PTCB EXAM PREP

The Most Comprehensive Study Guide
with 790 Questions,
5 Practice Tests,
Tips & Tricks, and Proven Strategies
for the Pharmacy Technician Certification

Table of Contents

What is the PTCB Exam?

Every time you pick up a prescription at a drugstore, you might wonder about the career behind the counter. You like the look of the job. Pharmacy technicians work in clean, bright environments, in the heart of a growing and secure industry—and they help connect people with the prescriptions they need for happier, healthier lives.

To earn this credential, you'll first need to pass the Pharmacy Technician Certification Board's (PTCB)® Pharmacy Technician Certification Exam (PTCE)®. If you could use a little extra insight into what this exam is like and how you can prepare for it, read on!

The Pharmacy Technician Certification Exam (PTCB) is a nationally recognized test that evaluates a candidate's knowledge and skills necessary to work as a pharmacy technician. Administered by the Pharmacy Technician Certification Board, the exam covers topics such as pharmacology, pharmacy law and regulations, medication safety, and quality assurance. Passing the PTCB exam grants certification, which can enhance job prospects, increase earning potential, and is often required by employers in the pharmacy field. This certification signifies a technician's ability to effectively assist pharmacists and ensure patient safety in pharmacy practices.

Introduction

Congratulations on taking the first step toward your Pharmacy Technician Certification. This guide is crafted to transform your preparation into a strategic, straightforward path to passing the PTCB Exam. Inside, you'll find everything required to not just pass but excel—thorough content reviews, rigorous practice tests, and proven strategies for success.

Embarking on this journey might seem daunting, but with the right tools at your disposal, achieving certification is within your reach. This book serves as your complete roadmap, guiding you through each essential topic and testing component with clarity and detail.

Prepare to dive deep into your studies with a resource designed to make complex information accessible and manageable. Success in the PTCB Exam opens doors to exciting career opportunities in pharmacy, and it all starts right here with your commitment to preparation.

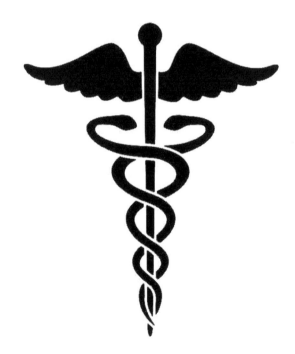

How to Use This Book

Follow these structured steps to optimize your preparation:

1. **Start with a Diagnostic Test:** Before diving into the material, take the initial diagnostic test included in the beginning of the book. This will help you identify your strengths and areas needing improvement, allowing you to focus your study time efficiently.

2. **Review the Study Material:** Each chapter of this book is dedicated to a specific section of the PTCB exam. Begin with the sections where you need the most review, as indicated by your diagnostic test results. Read through the detailed explanations and examples provided to solidify your understanding of key concepts.

3. **Utilize the Flashcards:** Enhance your retention of drug names, laws, and definitions by incorporating the flashcards into your study routine. Perfect for quick review sessions, these can be used anytime, anywhere. You'll find a link to download them at the end of this book.

4. **Practice with Exams:** After reviewing the chapters, test your knowledge with the practice exams. These are structured to emulate the actual PTCB exam, providing not just a test of knowledge but also a feel for the timing and pressure of the real test environment.

5. **Consult the PTCB Review Manual:** For deeper exploration of topics, refer to the included PDF review manual. It offers over 100 pages of comprehensive content review and additional exercises. The link to download the material is at the end of the book.

6. **Regular Review:** Consistency is key. Regularly revisit the chapters and materials to keep information fresh in your mind leading up to the exam date.

7. **Check Your Progress:** Use the answer keys and detailed explanations provided to gauge your progress. Understanding why answers are correct or incorrect will help you avoid common mistakes and fine-tune your knowledge.

Remember, persistence and a proactive approach to your studies will be your best tools for success.

Good luck!

Topics and Concepts You'll Discover on the PTCB Exam

The PTCB test focuses on the following topics:

- Medications (40%)
- Federal Requirements (12.5%)
- Patient Safety and Quality Assurance (26.25%)
- Order Entry and Processing (21.25%)

The Medications section is the most extensive and covers pharmaceutical classification, storage, contraindications, dose, interactions, and brand names versus generics. Examples of things you should be familiar with in this section include the active components in common drugs such as Zantac and the contraindications for a cholesterol medication such as Zocor. Brand and generic medicine names are among the most frequently asked exam questions. As a result, it is advisable to be familiar with the top 200 drugs encountered by the majority of pharmacy technicians.

Despite being the smallest component of the exam, many students find the Federal Requirements ideas the most challenging since they need you to understand and apply federal pharmacy legislation. You must understand federal requirements for controlled substances and prescriptions, how to handle and dispose of hazardous and non-hazardous goods, and what to do in the event of a recall.

The Patient Safety and Quality Assurance area evaluates your ability to give reasonable and cautious care to your patients. This section of the exam will assess your ability to detect and prevent errors, report unexpected events, and notify the pharmacist if an issue beyond the scope of your profession. To do well in this section, you should be familiar with cleanliness and hygiene standards, as well as medications that look and sound similar.

Order Processing and Entry will put your knowledge of compounded medications, syringes, and crucial pharmacy numbers (lot, expiration, and NDC) to the test. This part also covers common pharmaceutical calculations like ratio, portion, and conversion, so brush up on your pharmacy-related math skills before exam day.

Ten out of the 90 questions in the PTCB exam will be unscored. What exactly does this mean? It means that no matter how you answer the ten questions, they will have no bearing on your ultimate score. Unfortunately, you will not know which 10 questions are unscored, so you must give each question your utmost effort.

How to Pass the PTCB Exam

Did you know that seven dispensing pharmacies account for approximately 70% of the pharmacy business in the United States? Pharmacies are among the most common industries that employ pharmacy technologists.

Becoming a pharmacy technician gives you the opportunity to work with patients, pharmacists, and other healthcare professionals. The employment is frequently used as a first step toward a career as a pharmacist.

To become a pharmacy technician, you will most likely have to take and pass the PTCB exam. Many pupils begin to sweat as soon as they hear the word "exam." Fortunately, we are here to teach you more about how you may prepare for the PTCB and achieve the desired score the first time.

How to Prep for the PTCB Exam

Be Familiar With Topics That Will Appear On the Exam

Before taking any exam, you must be conversant with all of the topics presented. Because the PTCB exam needs a high level of specialized knowledge, you cannot simply show up on test day and rely on the fact that you are "good" at a specific subject, as you might have done on other general knowledge tests. If you have limited time to study for the PTCB, begin with reading the Medications part, which accounts for the majority of the exam.

Find the Study Method That Works Best for You

Everyone learns differently, therefore it's important to understand the study strategy that best suits you. Some people can read and absorb test preparation information, while others prefer a more "hands-on" approach, such as writing out definitions or generating tables and charts. According to studies, physically writing things down on paper improves memory recall. Creating physical flashcards and quizzing yourself can help you remember information more effectively than passively learning.

Take PTCB Practice Tests

Once you're confident in your understanding, attempt some practice questions. Practice exams are one of the finest indicators of how well-prepared you are, making them a vital tool for ensuring you pass the PTCB examination the first time. The PTCB offers official practice examinations for a charge, although there are also free PTCB practice tests available. If you are not using official exam preparation materials, be sure the website you are studying on is a high-quality resource that adheres to current test formatting and standards. Union Test Prep's PTCB practice test questions are designed to be the same style, difficulty level, and subject matter as those found on the actual PTCB exam, and they are an excellent resource to use while you prepare to take your test.

Use Pharmacy Exam Prep Material

In addition to a study guide, you may need extra exam preparation materials. These contain two major categories:

- Flashcards
- Practice exams

Let's start with the benefits of flashcards. Flashcard material is usually taken from a study guide and highlights crucial facts. The data should be brief and simple to remember. For instance, you could have placed the name of a medication on the front and a few vital data on the back, such as:

- Is it a controlled substance?
- What are common drug interactions?
- What drug dose or format does it come in?

Flash cards are important for two reasons. First, they encourage self-testing. From there, they provide an ideal baseline for learning and improvement.

If you only accurately recall 50% of your deck one week and 75% the next, you'll have a better idea of your progress. Flashcards can also help you identify areas that require more practice.

Ideally, for the PTCB exam, divide your flashcards into four groups based on the subjects stated above. As you practice each deck, you'll be able to select which courses to review in your study guide.

Practice examinations might help you prepare for test day. Using online practice examinations is undoubtedly the greatest approach to simulate test day. Online services such as Union Test Prep use test questions that are identical to those found on the actual exam. You can take many practice examinations to track your progress and decide passing grades.

Remember that taking a practice exam does not guarantee that you will cover the same subjects or questions on the actual test. You should use it in conjunction with the other tools mentioned above.

Practice With a Friend

One of the most difficult challenges is finding time and enthusiasm to study. Practising with a friend or family member helps you stay focused and motivated.

Practicing with a friend can also help you review flashcards and gain new perspectives on challenging concepts. It's even better if you can find a friend who is also preparing for the PTCB exam.

It's ideal to begin by going over the study guide together and discussing the facts you believe is most relevant or difficult to retain. After you've examined the study guide, begin creating flashcards for the subjects you've recognized as crucial.

Reviewing flashcards can make it easier to digest and comprehend information and essential concepts. Once you've mastered the flashcards, take a practice exam. This is one area that you should not attempt as a group. If you take a practice test with a friend, you may overlook areas that you struggle with separately.

Take Breaks

While it is beneficial to devote a significant amount of time and effort to your studies, you must also take breaks to allow your brain to relax and unwind. After all, you can't expect to perform optimally on exam day if your mind is fatigued and overwhelmed. Purposeful breaks of 5-60 minutes between study sessions can boost your energy and focus. "Purposeful" is the essential word here; aimless browsing on TikTok or Instagram will not provide the same advantages as stretching, calling a buddy, or taking a quick walk.

What To Expect on Exam Day

Taking a handful of practice examinations is the quickest approach to determine whether you are prepared for the PTCB exam. If your scores reflect your grasp of the exam materials, you may be ready to arrange your test.

Here is what you should prepare for on the day of the exam:
- Bring proof of identity (e.g., driver's license)
- Authorization to test letter or proof
- Leave electronics and personal belongings at home, in the car, or in the provided locker. Lockers are not available at all locations, so call the testing center ahead of time to confirm availability.
- Arrive early

The entire test is taken online, and you will not need pencils or calculators. Everything you need for the exam will be delivered to you. After completing the test, you will be given an unofficial score.

PTCB scores vary from 1000 to 1600, and you must score 1400 or more to pass. Your official score will be given within two to three weeks.

PTCB Diagnostic Test

Questions

Instructions:

- Answer all 25 multiple-choice questions.
- Each question has only one correct answer.
- This test is designed to assess your readiness across various topics related to pharmacy technician duties.
- Detailed explanations for each answer follow the test.

Pharmacology

Question 1:
What class of medication is commonly used to treat hypertension?
A) Anticoagulants
B) Beta-blockers
C) Antibiotics
D) Antivirals

Question 2:
Which medication is an example of a proton pump inhibitor?
A) Ranitidine
B) Omeprazole
C) Metformin
D) Ciprofloxacin

Pharmacy Law

Question 3:
Under the Controlled Substances Act, which schedule drug has the highest potential for abuse?
A) Schedule II
B) Schedule III
C) Schedule IV
D) Schedule V

Medication Safety

Question 4:
Which of the following is a critical check before dispensing medication?
A) Checking the drug's color
B) Verifying patient's name and date of birth
C) Assessing the taste of the medication
D) Confirming the price of the drug

Quality Assurance

Question 5:
What is the primary purpose of medication reconciliation?
A) To ensure that prices are accurate
B) To document the refusal of medication
C) To verify all medications are correctly prescribed and administered
D) To check the expiration dates of drugs on the shelf

Medication Order and Prescription Interpretation

Question 6:
The abbreviation "q.d." on a prescription stands for:
A) Four times a day
B) Once daily
C) Every other day
D) As needed

Drug Classifications

Question 7:
Which type of drug is used to lower cholesterol?
A) Antipsychotic
B) Antipyretic
C) Statin
D) Antitussive

Sterile Compounding

Question 8:
What is the primary concern when preparing IV admixtures?
A) Flavor
B) Cost
C) Sterility
D) Color

Pharmacy Calculations

Question 9:
How many milliliters of a 1% solution can be made from 5 grams of solute?
A) 500 ml
B) 50 ml
C) 5 ml
D) 1000 ml

Inventory Management

Question 10:
What is a primary objective of inventory management in a pharmacy?
A) Maximizing shelf space
B) Minimizing medication cost
C) Maintaining adequate stock levels
D) Displaying promotional items

Non-Sterile Compounding

Question 11:
What is the key factor in choosing an excipient for a non-sterile compounded medication?
A) Taste
B) Solubility
C) Color
D) Cost

Billing and Reimbursement

Question 12:
What is a primary purpose of the National Drug Code (NDC) on prescription drugs?
A) Tracking inventory
B) Identifying drugs uniquely
C) Promoting drugs
D) Regulating prices

Federal Requirements

Question 13:
Which federal agency regulates the sale of medications that have the potential for abuse?
A) FDA
B) DEA
C) FCC
D) USDA

Patient Safety and Quality Assurance

Question 14:
What is the role of a pharmacy technician in promoting patient safety?
A) Managing the pharmacy's budget
B) Ensuring accurate dispensing and labeling of medications
C) Marketing new medications
D) Setting prices for medications

Order Entry and Processing

Question 15:
What information is essential when processing a prescription order?
A) Patient's favorite color
B) Time of day
C) Patient's medication allergies
D) Patient's income level

Pharmaceutical Calculations

Question 16:
Calculate the amount of dextrose in grams in 500 mL of D10W.
A) 5 grams
B) 50 grams
C) 10 grams
D) 100 grams

Pharmacology

Question 17:
Which medication is NOT considered an anticoagulant?
A) Warfarin
B) Heparin
C) Ibuprofen
D) Enoxaparin

Medication Administration

Question 18:
Which route of medication administration is used for insulin delivery?
A) Oral
B) Subcutaneous
C) Intravenous
D) Topical

Clinical Use of Drugs

Question 19:
What is the primary use of albuterol?
A) Pain relief
B) Blood clot prevention
C) Asthma symptom control
D) Blood pressure reduction

Pharmacy Ethics

Question 20:
It is unethical for a pharmacy technician to:
A) Maintain patient confidentiality
B) Accept gifts from pharmaceutical representatives
C) Provide patient counseling
D) Dispense prescribed medications

Community Pharmacy

Question 21:
Which is a common task for a pharmacy technician in a community pharmacy setting?
A) Prescribing medications
B) Conducting health screenings
C) Managing prescription refills
D) Performing surgery

Hospital Pharmacy

Question 22:
What is the role of a pharmacy technician in a hospital setting regarding medication distribution?
A) Deciding on patient medication plans
B) Preparing and delivering medications to nursing units
C) Performing medical procedures
D) Diagnosing patient conditions

Drug Interactions

Question 23:
Which of the following could potentially cause a serious interaction with warfarin?
A) Vitamin K
B) Vitamin C
C) Vitamin D
D) Vitamin E

Dosage Calculations

Question 24:
How many mL of a 2% lidocaine solution contains 200 mg of lidocaine?
A) 10 mL
B) 5 mL
C) 20 mL
D) 100 mL

Pharmaceutical Compounding

Question 25:
What is the primary reason for compounding a medication for a patient?
A) To create a medication that is commercially unavailable
B) To increase the pharmacy's revenue
C) To make the medication taste worse
D) To comply with pharmaceutical advertising

Below is a table for you to record your answers. After completing the test, use it to check whether your responses were correct and to review the explanations provided for each answer.

Question Number	Correct Answer	Your Answer	Explanation
1			
2			
3			
4			
5			
6			
7			
8			
9			
10			
11			
12			
13			
14			
15			
16			
17			
18			
19			
20			
21			
22			
23			
24			
25			

Detailed Answers and Explanations

Question 1:

Correct Answer: B - Beta-blockers are used to manage hypertension by reducing heart rate and the force of heart contractions.

Question 2:

Correct Answer: B - Omeprazole is a proton pump inhibitor that reduces stomach acid production.

Question 3:

Correct Answer: A - Schedule II drugs have a high potential for abuse and may lead to severe psychological or physical dependence.

Question 4:

Correct Answer: B - Verifying the patient's identity (name and date of birth) is crucial for safety.

Question 5:

Correct Answer: C - Medication reconciliation ensures all medications are correctly prescribed, administered, and documented.

Question 6:

Correct Answer: B - "q.d." is Latin for "quaque die," meaning once a day.

Question 7:

Correct Answer: C - Statins are used to lower cholesterol levels in the blood.

Question 8:

Correct Answer: C - Ensuring sterility is crucial in the preparation of IV admixtures to prevent infections.

Question 9:

Correct Answer: A - 500 ml of solution is needed for 5 grams of solute to make a 1% solution (1 gram per 100 ml).

Question 10:

Correct Answer: C - The main goal is to maintain adequate stock levels to meet patient needs without overstocking.

Question 11:

Correct Answer: B - Solubility is crucial for ensuring the active ingredients are effectively absorbed.

Question 12:

Correct Answer: B - The NDC uniquely identifies all drugs marketed in the U.S.

Question 13:

Correct Answer: B - The Drug Enforcement Administration (DEA) regulates the sale of controlled substances.

Question 14:

Correct Answer: B - Pharmacy technicians ensure medications are accurately dispensed and labeled, crucial for patient safety.

Question 15:

Correct Answer: C - Knowing a patient's medication allergies is essential to avoid harmful reactions.

Question 16:

Correct Answer: B - D10W means 10% dextrose, so 500 mL contains 50 grams of dextrose (10 grams per 100 mL).

Question 17:

Correct Answer: C - Ibuprofen is a nonsteroidal anti-inflammatory drug (NSAID), not an anticoagulant.

Question 18:

Correct Answer: B - Insulin is typically administered subcutaneously.

Question 19:

Correct Answer: C - Albuterol is primarily used to treat and prevent bronchospasm in people with asthma.

Question 20:

Correct Answer: B - Accepting gifts from pharmaceutical reps can lead to conflicts of interest and is generally considered unethical in pharmacy practice.

Question 21:

Correct Answer: C - Managing prescription refills is a common responsibility of pharmacy technicians in community pharmacies.

Question 22:

Correct Answer: B - Pharmacy technicians in hospitals often prepare and deliver medications to various hospital departments.

Question 23:

Correct Answer: A - Vitamin K can counteract the anticoagulant effects of warfarin, leading to potential clotting issues.

Question 24:

Correct Answer: A - A 2% solution means 2 grams per 100 mL, or 200 mg per 10 mL.

Question 25:

Correct Answer: A - Compounding is often necessary when a specific medication is needed that is not available commercially or needs to be customized for a patient's specific needs (e.g., allergies, pediatric dosages).

This diagnostic test is designed to help you identify which areas need further review. Don't worry, though—by the end of this book, you'll have access to 5 practice tests, 380 flashcards, a comprehensive PTCB Review Manual PDF of over 100 pages and a PDF of PTCB Pharmacy Calculations with all the formulas to fully prepare you for your exam.

Master Drug Knowledge for the PTCB Exam

Studying for the Pharmacy Technician Certification Board (PTCB) exam is a major task, with the need to learn a wide selection of generic and brand-name medications that might be intimidating. The use of mnemonics, ingenious memory devices meant to aid with information retention, has shown to be a beneficial method for many pupils. Today, we'll look at some important pharmacological mnemonics that could give you a significant advantage on PTCB exam day.

1. ACE Inhibitors: "A 'PRIL' in need is a friend indeed!"

Angiotensin-Converting Enzyme (ACE) inhibitors are a class of drugs used to treat hypertension and heart failure. These medicines are distinguished by their names, which typically finish in "-pril." ACE inhibitors include lisinopril, available under the brand names Prinivil and Zestril, enalapril (brand name Vasotec), and ramipril, also known as Altace. The mnemonic to remember here is that 'pril' sounds like April - a month, or even a helpful assistant. So, whenever you come across these meds, think of them as your trustworthy friend, 'Pril,' who is always ready to aid when it comes to dealing with hypertension and heart failure.

2. Beta Blockers: "Oh 'LOL', it's time to relax!"

Beta-blockers, also known as beta-adrenergic blocking medications, are another class of pharmaceuticals used to treat cardiovascular diseases such as hypertension, angina, and arrhythmias. The link between these drugs is that their names frequently finish in "-lol." This is the case with metoprolol, which is sold under the brand names Lopressor and Toprol-XL, atenolol, also known as Tenormin, and propranolol, also known as Inderal. The mnemonic here is the online slang phrase 'LOL,' which stands for 'laugh out loud.' These 'lol' medications work to lower your blood pressure, alleviate chest pain, and regulate your heart rhythm, so imagine your heart 'laughing out loud' in relief. So, when you face a Beta Blocker, remember the soothing effect of a good, hearty chuckle - and then relax!

3. Statins: "Remember, it's no 'STATIN' the fact you need to lower your cholesterol."

Statins, also known as HMG-CoA reductase inhibitors, are medications that help decrease cholesterol levels in the blood, potentially preventing heart disease and stroke. They accomplish this by inhibiting the enzyme that your liver uses to produce cholesterol. These drugs often end in "-statin," such as atorvastatin (Lipitor), rosuvastatin (Crestor), and simvastatin (Zocor). The mnemonic here is "statin," which sounds like "stating," so consider these treatments as "stating" the importance of cholesterol reduction. Every time you see a pill ending in '-statin,' remember it's used to manage cholesterol levels, underscoring the critical role these medications play in cardiovascular health.

4. Proton Pump Inhibitors: "In a 'ZOLE', there's less acid."

Proton pump inhibitors (PPIs) are a class of medications that cause a significant and long-lasting reduction in stomach acid production. They are among the world's best-selling medications and are used to treat illnesses characterized by high stomach acid levels, such as ulcers, gastroesophageal reflux disease (GERD), and Zollinger-Ellison syndrome. Most PPI names end in "-azole," such as omeprazole (Prilosec), pantoprazole (Protonix), and esomeprazole (Nexium). The mnemonic "zole" sounds like "hole," and it is simple to imagine a "hole" where the excess acid has been eliminated. This image of a 'zole' or 'hole' with less acid can serve as a quick reminder that "-azole" drugs are used to reduce acidity in your stomach.

5. Glucocorticoids: "The 'SONE' is shining, you feel strong."

Glucocorticoids are steroid hormones that play an important role in a variety of physiological processes, including stress management, immunological response, and inflammation control. Glucocorticoids also help the body metabolize carbohydrates, proteins, and fats. Prednisone, hydrocortisone, and dexamethasone are some examples of medications that finish in "-sone." The mnemonic here is "sone," which sounds similar to "sun." These'sone' medicines provide strength by reducing inflammation and suppressing overactive immune responses, much way the sun provides light and vitality. So, anytime you come across these meds, imagine a bright, sunny day when you feel strong, healthy, and free of inflammation.

6. Antifungals: "FUNgal infections can't survive in the 'AZOLE'."

Antifungal medications are a type of drug that targets and eliminates fungal organisms, hence relieving infections. Many antifungal drugs finish in "-azole," including ketoconazole, fluconazole, and itraconazole. Here, the mnemonic is 'azole,' which you might humorously recall as "a hole." Fungi cannot have fun ('FUNgal') in a 'azole' or "a hole". This term serves as a rapid reminder that 'azole' medications are antifungal agents, ready to create an environment in which fungi cannot live.

7. Benzodiazepines: "It's 'ZOLAM' quiet, time for rest."

Benzodiazepines are a class of psychoactive medications that are commonly used to treat anxiety, insomnia, seizures, alcohol withdrawal, and muscle relaxation. These medications function by increasing the effect of the neurotransmitter gamma-aminobutyric acid (GABA), resulting in sedative, sleep-inducing, anxiolytic, anticonvulsant, and muscle relaxant effects. Many benzodiazepines finish in "-zolam" or "-zepam," including alprazolam (Xanax), lorazepam (Ativan), and diazepam (Valium). The mnemonic to remember here is "zolam," which translates to "so calm." When you think of these medicines, imagine a serene scene with 'zolam' silence, which represents the tranquillity and slumber that benzodiazepines can bring.

8. Phosphodiesterase-5 (PDE5) inhibitors: "'AFIL' of love!"

Phosphodiesterase-5 (PDE5) inhibitors are a type of medication used largely to treat erectile dysfunction and, in certain situations, pulmonary arterial hypertension. Examples ending in "-afil" include sildenafil (brand name Viagra), tadalafil (Cialis), and vardenafil (Levitra). To assist remember this pharmacological class, consider "afil" to be a phonetic play on the words "a feel" or even "affection". It's a clever approach to link these pharmaceuticals to their fundamental purpose of sexual health and the heart, which are both symbolically and medically associated with love.

9. Angiotensin II Receptor Blockers (ARBs): "Angiotensin ends in 'sartan' in the 'ARB'or."

Angiotensin II receptor blockers (ARBs) are drugs that inhibit the action of angiotensin II, allowing blood vessels to relax and widen, resulting in a drop in blood pressure. These are commonly used to treat excessive blood pressure and heart failure. Most of these medicines end in "-sartan," including losartan (Cozaar), valsartan (Diovan), and irbesartan (Avapro). To help remember this, imagine "sartan" sounding like a "sailor's tan," and picturing these medications in the 'ARB'or (harbor), ready to set sail and fight high blood pressure.

10. 5-alpha reductase inhibitors: "'STERIDE' off the DHT."

5-alpha reductase inhibitors are generally used to treat benign prostate hyperplasia (BPH) and male pattern baldness. various drugs work by preventing the conversion of testosterone to dihydrotestosterone (DHT), a hormone that can contribute to various disorders. Drugs in this category frequently end with "-steride," such as finasteride (Proscar, Propecia) and dutasteride (Avodart). As a mnemonic, consider "steride" to be a play on the term "stride." Imagine these medications striding or marching forward, determined to eliminate the undesirable DHT.

Mastering drug classifications for the PTCB exam may appear difficult at first. However, using inventive mnemonics can significantly improve your capacity to remember and understand these classifications. However, memorizing the topic matter is only one aspect of the preparation process.

Regular practice examinations are also a vital part of your study schedule. They not only strengthen your understanding and remembrance of the information, but they also help you familiarize yourself with the structure and schedule of the actual exam. Practice exams allow you to monitor your learning progress, identify any issues that need more focus, and gain confidence as you see your results gradually improve.

Top 200 Drugs on the PTCB

The Pharmacy Technician Certification Board (PTCB) exam is the final step toward becoming a qualified pharmacy technician. The credential is your ticket to a bright future in pharmacy, so this test is critical.

The PTCB exam can be difficult, thus preparation is essential for success. To achieve the desired score, you must maintain a hard study regimen. To get you started, these are the top 200 medicines you're likely to encounter on the PTCB exam. They are organized by medicine kind, including brand and generic names, and are presented in a chart below. Familiarizing yourself with the top 200 medications and their uses will help you score well on the PTCB exam.

5-Alpha Reductase Inhibitor

5-Alpha reductase inhibitors are a type of medication used to treat enlarged prostate glands. (It should be noted that these medications are not licensed for treating prostate cancer.) They can also treat hair loss, such as male pattern baldness.

Avodart (dutasteride)

Proscar (finasteride) is an oral medication that can be used alone or in conjunction with other prostate therapies.

ACE inhibitor

Angiotensin-converting enzyme (ACE) inhibitors relax the arteries and veins, which can assist to reduce blood pressure. They function by inhibiting the formation of angiotensin II, a chemical that narrows blood arteries, by specific enzymes in the body.

- Aceon (perindopril)
- Altace (ramipril)
- Epaned (enalapril)
- Norvasc (amlodipine)
- Prinivil (lisinopril)
- Qbrelis (lisinopril)
- Vasotec (enalapril)

Alpha-1 Blocker

Alpha-1 adrenergic receptor antagonists, often known as alpha-blockers, interact with type 1 alpha-adrenergic receptors. This binding prevents smooth muscle contraction, which can help treat hypertension and benign prostatic hypertrophy.

- Cardura (doxazosin)
- Hytrin (terazosin)
- Uroxatral (alfuzosin)

Antipyretic Analgesics

Antipyretic analgesics provide pain relief while also lowering raised body temperatures caused by fever.

- Fioricet (acetaminophen, butalbital, and caffeine)
- Night Time (acetaminophen and diphenhydramine)
- Percocet (acetaminophen and oxycodone)
- Pyridium (phenazopyridine)
- Tylenol (acetaminophen)
- Vicodin (acetaminophen and hydrocodone, an opioid)

Anti-Gout Medications

These drugs treat the prevalent inflammatory arthritis associated with gout. Allopurinols reduce the amount of uric acid the body produces, whereas colchicine relieves gout discomfort.

- Colcrys (colchicine)
- Mitigare (colchicine)

- Zyloprim (allopurinol)

Anti-Malarial Medications

In some parts of the world, anti-malarial drugs both treat and prevent malaria infection.

- Plaquenil (hydroxychloroquine)

Anti-Migraine Medications

These drugs work by targeting the brain's trigeminovascular system. They relieve migraines and cluster headaches.

- Relpax (eletriptan)
- Imitrex (sumatriptan)
- Zomig (zolmitriptan)

Antibiotics and Antibacterial Medications

On the PTCB exam, you will very probably face a variety of medications used to treat bacterial infections such as pneumonia, bronchitis, and disorders of the ears, nose, throat, and other parts of the body.

Penicillin, discovered by Dr. Alexander Fleming in 1928, is a beta-lactam that inhibits the synthesis of peptidoglycan molecules, which help bacteria form strong bonds. Some of the medications on this list, such as Flagyl, also work as anti-protozoal agents.

- Adoxa (doxycycline)
- Amoxil Trimox (amoxicillin)
- Augmentin (amoxicillin and clavulanic acid)
- Avelox (moxifloxacin)
- Bactroban (mupirocin)
- Biaxin (clarithromycin)
- Ceftin (cefuroxime)
- Cipro (ciprofloxacin)
- Cleocin (clindamycin)
- Flagyl (metronidazole)
- Keflex (cephalexin)
- Levaquin (levofloxacin)
- Macrobid Macrodantin (nitrofurantoin)
- Omicef (cefdinir)
- PC Pen VK (penicillin)
- Pen V (penicillin)
- Proquin (ciprofloxacin)
- Sumycin Ala-Tet Brodspec (tetracycline)

- Vibramycin (doxycycline)
- Zithromax (azithromycin)

Anti-Cancer Medications

Pemetrexed and bevacizumab medications are frequently used as the first-line treatment for metastatic cancer with no gene alterations. Common forms include ovarian, non-squamous, and non-small-cell lung cancer.

- Alimta (pemetrexed)
- Avastin (bevacizumab)

Anticoagulant Medications

Anticoagulant drugs act by disrupting the processes that lead to the formation of blood clots. These medications are used as a prophylactic measure for those who are at high risk of blood clots, which can cause dangerous diseases such as heart attacks and strokes.

- Coumadin (warfarin)
- Eliquis (apixaban)
- Fragmin (dalteparin)
- Heparin Sodium (heparin)
- Lovenox (enoxaparin)
- Pradaxa (dabigatran)
- Xarelto (rivaroxaban)

Anticonvulsant Medications

Anticonvulsant or anti-seizure drugs are commonly used to treat epilepsy and other chronic seizure disorders. They are also utilized for patients who have recently had brain surgery or another operation involving the central nervous system. They function by reducing aberrant electrical activity in the brain.

- Depacon Depakote (valproate sodium)
- Dilantin (phenytoin)
- Keppra (levetiracetam)
- Lamictal (lamotrigine)
- Lyrica (pregabalin)
- Neurontin (gabapentin)

Antidepressants

Antidepressants are medications that help to prevent or cure clinical depression. Most antidepressants operate by restoring equilibrium or increasing the production of certain chemicals in the brain, such as serotonin. They can also help treat other illnesses, such as generalized anxiety disorder or obsessive-compulsive disorder.

- Celexa (citalopram)

- Desyrel (trazodone)
- Elavil (amitriptyline)
- Lexapro (escitalopram)
- Luvox (fluvoxamine)
- Pamelor (nortriptyline)
- Paxil (paroxetine)
- Prozac Sarafem (fluoxetine)
- Tofranil (imipramine)
- Vanatrip (amitriptyline)
- Zoloft (sertraline)

Antidiabetic Medications

Antidiabetics are a type of medication that treats the symptoms of diabetes, particularly type 2 diabetes, by reducing high blood sugar levels in a variety of methods. For example, glyburide and sitagliptin cause the pancreas to release more insulin into the bloodstream. Metformin-containing medications help the body handle insulin more effectively.

- Amaryl (glimepiride)
- DiaBeta (glyburide)
- Glucophage (metformin)
- Glucotrol (glipizide)
- HumuLIN (insulin isophane)
- HumaLOG (insulin lispro)
- Invokana (canagliflozin)
- Januvia (sitagliptin)
- Lantus (insulin glargine)
- Levemir (insulin detemir)
- NovoLog (insulin aspart)
- Reglan (metoclopramide)
- Saxenda Victoza (liraglutide)

Antiemetic Medications

Antiemetic drugs are used to relieve nausea and vomiting. Common treatments include those for motion nausea, viral or bacterial illnesses (such as stomach flu), pregnancy, and the side effects of surgery or chemotherapy.

- Kytril Sancuso (granisetron)
- Zofran (ondansetron)

Antifungal Medications

Antifungal drugs eliminate or inhibit the growth of fungal infections in the body. While fungal infections can affect anybody, they can be particularly dangerous for patients with autoimmune disorders such as lupus or AIDS, cancer, or who have undergone stem cell transplants.

- Diflucan (fluconazole)
- Lotrisone (clotrimazole and betamethasone)
- Nizoral Topical (ketoconazole)

Antihistamines

Antihistamines, as the name implies, prevent the effects of histamine, a chemical released by your body in response to a hazardous infection. Histamine causes blood vessels to dilate and the skin to bulge in order to protect the body. Antihistamines stop the reaction when it occurs as a result of an allergy.

- Tussionex PennKinetic (chlorpheniramine and hydrocodone)

Anti-inflammatory Drugs

Prednisone and other anti-inflammatory drugs help to manage inflammation in the joints and organs. Anti-inflammatory medications such as hydrocortisone and triamcinolone alleviate pain caused by inflammation of the skin. Nonsteroidal anti-inflammatory medications (NSAIDs) are commonly used to treat headaches and mild injuries.

- Advil (ibuprofen)
- Ala-Cort (hydrocortisone)
- Aleve (naproxen)
- Aristocort (triamcinolone)
- Cataflam (diclofenac)
- Celebrex (celecoxib)
- Deltasone (prednisone)
- Flo-Pred (prednisolone)
- Mobic (meloxicam)
- Rayos (prednisone)
- Relafen (nabumetone)

Anti-insomnia Medications

Anti-insomnia drugs operate by reducing brain activity, allowing people to fall and remain asleep more easily.

- Ambien (zolpidem)
- Lunesta (eszopiclone)
- Sonata (zaleplon)

Antiretroviral Medications

Antiretroviral drugs, including those containing valganciclovir, are designed to delay the progression of HIV or hepatitis C.

- Atripla (emtricitabine, tenofovir, and efavirenz)
- Isentress (raltegravir)
- Sovaldi (sofosbuvir)
- Valcyte (valganciclovir)
- Zovirax (acyclovir)

Asthma and Bronchitis Medications

Beta-2 agonists are drugs that alter the epinephrine molecule to facilitate specific contact with beta-2 receptors on bronchial muscles. They are used to treat bronchial asthma and chronic obstructive pulmonary disorder (COPD).

- Advair (salmeterol and fluticasone)
- Combivent Respimat (albuterol and ipratropium)
- ProAir (albuterol)
- Proventil (albuterol)
- Singulair (montelukast)
- Ventolin (albuterol)

Attention Deficit Disorder

ADHD is one of the most prevalent neurodevelopmental diseases in children. Medications containing methylphenidate are central nervous system stimulants used to treat ADHD and other illnesses such as narcolepsy.

- Concerta (methylphenidate)
- Ritalin (methylphenidate)

Benzodiazepines

Benzodiazepines are used to treat severe anxiety, such as panic attacks, and sleeplessness. They function by urging the brain to release gamma-aminobutyric acid, a neurotransmitter that reduces nervous system activity.

- Ativan (lorazepam)
- Klonopin (clonazepam)
- Restoril (temazepam)
- Valium (diazepam)
- Xanax (alprazolam)

Beta-Blockers and Nitrate Medications

Beta-blockers are a class of medications that reduce heart rate by inhibiting chemicals such as adrenaline. Nitrate drugs improve blood flow, which reduces heart stress.

- Coreg (carvedilol)
- Imdur (isosorbide mononitrate)
- Lopressor (metoprolol)
- NitroStat Sublingual (nitroglycerin)
- Tenormin (atenolol)
- Zebeta (bisoprolol)

Birth Control

There are numerous types of medications used for female birth control. The hormones that contribute to an egg's complete development each month are most affected. Yaz is the most likely candidate you will encounter on the PTCB exam.

- Yaz (ethinyl estradiol and drospirenone)

Blood Pressure Medications

Every year, high blood pressure, also known as hypertension, causes more than 670,000 fatalities in the United States.

Hydralazine-containing medications lower blood pressure by relaxing blood arteries, which reduces the workload of the heart.

Clopidogrel-containing medications help thin the blood, which lowers blood vessel pressure.

- Apresoline (hydralazine)
- Plavix (clopidogrel)

Bone Health

Bisphosphonates, including those containing zoledronic acid, can help treat Paget's disease, multiple myeloma, and a variety of bone malignancies.

- Actonel (risedronate)
- Boniva (ibandronate)
- Fosamax (alendronate)
- Reclast (zoledronic acid)
- Zometa (zoledronic acid)

Brain Disorder Medications

Many medications are intended to alleviate the symptoms of neurological illnesses such as Alzheimer's and Parkinson's. Acetylcholinesterase inhibitors, such as donepezil, prevent the breakdown of the neurotransmitter acetylcholine into acetate and choline.

- Aricept (donepezil)

- Clozaril (clozapine)
- Cogentin (benztropine)
- Haldol (haloperidol)
- Inbrija Dopar Larodopa (levodopa)
- Requip (ropinirole)
- Risperdal (risperidone)
- Seroquel (quetiapine)
- Stalevo 50 (levodopa, carbidopa, and entacapone)
- Zyprexa (olanzapine)

Cholesterol Medications

High cholesterol can cause a variety of health concerns. Drugs containing ezetimibe, an antihyperlipidemic, assist decrease blood cholesterol levels. Triglyceride-lowering drugs contain omega-3 fatty acids.

- Altoprev (lovastatin)
- Antara (fenofibrate)
- Crestor (rosuvastatin)
- Lipitor (atorvastatin)
- Lopid (gemfibrozil)
- Lovaza (omega-3 fatty acids)
- Mevacor (lovastatin)
- Pravachol (pravastatin)
- Niaspan (niacin)
- TriCor (fenofibrate)
- Zetia (ezetimibe)
- Zocor (simvastatin)

Common Cold/Flu Symptom Medications

Aspirin and other antipyretic drugs help to lower fever. Antitussive expectorants, such as those containing dextromethorphan, ease coughs, but they are not meant to treat chronic coughs caused by asthma, emphysema, or long-term smoking.

- Bayer (aspirin)
- Bufferin (aspirin)
- Ecotrin (aspirin)
- Robitussin (dextromethorphan and guaifenesin)
- Tamiflu (oseltamivir)

Disinfectant/Antiseptics and Topical Anesthetic

Topical antiseptics can be used to disinfect the skin after an injury or prior to an injection or surgery. Lidocaine is a topical anesthetic that relieves pain by inhibiting signals from the skin's nerve endings.

- BetaSept (chlorhexidine)
- ChloraPrep (chlorhexidine)
- Lidoderm (lidocaine)

Erectile Dysfunction

Erectile dysfunction drugs operate by relaxing the muscles and arteries of the penis, increasing blood flow and allowing for erections. Tadalafil-containing drugs can also help treat an enlarged prostate.

- Cialis (tadalafil)
- Levitra (vardenafil)
- Viagra (sildenafil)

Estrogen Modulators/Replacements

Medications containing raloxifene, for example, can help prevent or treat symptoms caused by low estrogen levels during menopause. These include "hot flashes" and the onset of osteoporosis.

- Evista (raloxifene)
- Premarin (conjugated estrogens)

Gastrointestinal Medications

Antispasmodic and anticholinergic medicines, such as dicyclomine and tiotropium, alleviate muscle spasms in the gastrointestinal system. They accomplish this by inhibiting the activity of several natural chemicals in the body. They are commonly used to treat irritable bowel syndrome.

Other drugs, such as those containing famotidine, work as H2-receptor antagonists to cure or prevent ulcers. Those containing lactulose and senna are categorized as laxatives and are intended to alleviate constipation.

- AcipHex (rabeprazole)
- Bentyl (dicyclomine)
- Constulose (lactulose)
- Ex-Lax (senna)
- Pepcid (famotidine)
- Prevacid (lansoprazole)
- Prilosec (omeprazole)
- Nexium (esomeprazole)

- Senna Lax (senna)
- Spiriva (tiotropium)
- Vesicare (solifenacin)
- Zantac (ranitidine)

Kidney Disease Medications

Cinacalcet-containing medications are used to treat secondary hyperparathyroidism in people with chronic renal disease. Furosemide-containing medications are diuretics that can alleviate fluid retention and organ edema.

- Sensipar (cinacalcet)
- Lasix (furosemide)

Immunosuppressants

Immunosuppressants inhibit the immune system's natural response to a variety of disorders, ranging from organ rejection after transplantation to severe inflammatory diseases such as psoriasis, psoriatic arthritis, and multiple sclerosis.

- Enbrel (etanercept)
- Gilenya (fingolimod)
- Neoral (cyclosporin)
- Otrexup (methotrexate)
- SandIMMUNE (cyclosporin)

Monoclonal Antibodies

Monoclonal antibody treatment is an infusion or injection aimed to combat several illnesses, including COVID-19, osteoporosis, inflammatory disorders, and some malignancies.

- Herceptin (trastuzumab)
- Prolia (denosumab)
- Remicade (infliximab)
- Stelara (ustekinumab)
- Xgeva (denosumab)
- Xolair (omalizumab)

Muscle Relaxants

Muscular relaxants work by slowing down brain and nerve processes that control muscular tone, causing the muscles to relax.

- Carbacot (methocarbamol)
- Lioresal (baclofen)
- Robaxin (methocarbamol)
- Zanaflex (tizanidine)

Opiate Narcotics/Analgesics

Opioids are highly strong opioids used to relieve severe pain. Certain drugs, such as those containing methadone, can be used to treat opioid addiction.

- Duragesic (fentanyl)
- Methadose (methadone)
- Ultram (tramadol)

Summary of the Top 200 Drugs for the PTCB Exam

Brand Name	Generic Name	Drug Classification
Lipitor	atorvastatin	Statin
Zestril	lisinopril	ACE inhibitor
Norvasc	amlodipine	Calcium channel blocker
Synthroid	levothyroxine	Thyroid medication
Plavix	clopidogrel	Antiplatelet agent
Nexium	esomeprazole	Proton pump inhibitor
Advair Diskus	fluticasone/salmeterol	Bronchodilator + steroid
Crestor	rosuvastatin	Statin
Cymbalta	duloxetine	SNRI antidepressant
Vyvanse	lisdexamfetamine	CNS stimulant
Lasix	furosemide	Diuretic
Coumadin	warfarin	Anticoagulant
Lantus	insulin glargine	Insulin
Neurontin	gabapentin	Antiepileptic/Antineuralgic
Zoloft	sertraline	SSRI antidepressant
ProAir HFA	albuterol	Bronchodilator
Augmentin	amoxicillin/clavulanate	Antibiotic
Ambien	zolpidem	Sedative
Singulair	montelukast	Leukotriene receptor antagonist
Metoprolol Tartrate	metoprolol	Beta-blocker
Seroquel XR	quetiapine	Atypical antipsychotic
Diovan	valsartan	ARB (Angiotensin receptor blocker)
Viagra	sildenafil	Erectile dysfunction treatment
Zocor	simvastatin	Statin
Flexeril	cyclobenzaprine	Muscle relaxant
Concerta	methylphenidate	CNS stimulant (for ADHD)
Tamiflu	oseltamivir	Antiviral
Mobic	meloxicam	NSAID

Brand Name	Generic Name	Drug Classification
Premarin	conjugated estrogens	Estrogen replacement
Bactrim DS	sulfamethoxazole/trimethoprim	Antibiotic
Effexor XR	venlafaxine	SNRI antidepressant
Toprol XL	metoprolol succinate	Beta-blocker
Glucophage	metformin	Antidiabetic
Prozac	fluoxetine	SSRI antidepressant
Celebrex	celecoxib	NSAID
Klonopin	clonazepam	Benzodiazepine
Abilify	aripiprazole	Atypical antipsychotic
OxyContin	oxycodone	Opioid analgesic
Diflucan	fluconazole	Antifungal
Paxil	paroxetine	SSRI antidepressant
Prilosec	omeprazole	Proton pump inhibitor
Lyrica	pregabalin	Antiepileptic/Antineuralgic
Xanax	alprazolam	Benzodiazepine
Spiriva	tiotropium	Anticholinergic bronchodilator
Januvia	sitagliptin	DPP-4 inhibitor (Antidiabetic)
Tricor	fenofibrate	Antihyperlipidemic
Actos	pioglitazone	Antidiabetic
Levaquin	levofloxacin	Antibiotic
Nasonex	mometasone	Corticosteroid (nasal spray)
Benicar	olmesartan	ARB (Angiotensin receptor blocker)
Ultram	tramadol	Opioid analgesic
Fosamax	alendronate	Bisphosphonate (for osteoporosis)
Suboxone	buprenorphine/naloxone	Opioid dependence treatment
Insulin Regular	humulin R, novolin R	Insulin
Lunesta	eszopiclone	Sedative
Lotensin	benazepril	ACE inhibitor
Avapro	irbesartan	ARB (Angiotensin receptor blocker)
Advil/Motrin	ibuprofen	NSAID
Depakote	divalproex	Antiepileptic
Strattera	atomoxetine	NRI (for ADHD)
Valtrex	valacyclovir	Antiviral
Aleve	naproxen	NSAID
Vytorin	ezetimibe/simvastatin	Antihyperlipidemic
Cipro	ciprofloxacin	Antibiotic
Coreg	carvedilol	Beta-blocker
Keppra	levetiracetam	Antiepileptic
Claritin	loratadine	Antihistamine

Brand Name	Generic Name	Drug Classification
Flonase	fluticasone (nasal)	Corticosteroid (nasal spray)
Zetia	ezetimibe	Antihyperlipidemic
Risperdal	risperidone	Atypical antipsychotic
Tylenol	acetaminophen	Analgesic/Antipyretic
Altace	ramipril	ACE inhibitor
Zyprexa	olanzapine	Atypical antipsychotic
Wellbutrin	bupropion	Antidepressant
Desyrel	trazodone	Antidepressant
Accupril	quinapril	ACE inhibitor
Plendil	felodipine	Calcium channel blocker
Evista	raloxifene	SERM (Selective estrogen receptor modulator)
Imdur	isosorbide mononitrate	Nitrate (for angina)
Adderall XR	amphetamine/dextroamphetamine	CNS stimulant (for ADHD)
Bystolic	nebivolol	Beta-blocker
Lanoxin	digoxin	Cardiac glycoside
Hyzaar	losartan/hydrochlorothiazide	ARB + Diuretic
Catapres	clonidine	Alpha-2 agonist
Atarax	hydroxyzine	Antihistamine
Geodon	ziprasidone	Atypical antipsychotic
Cardizem	diltiazem	Calcium channel blocker
Elavil	amitriptyline	Tricyclic antidepressant
Amaryl	glimepiride	Sulfonylurea (Antidiabetic)
Tenormin	atenolol	Beta-blocker
Dilantin	phenytoin	Antiepileptic
Maxalt	rizatriptan	Triptan (for migraines)
Glucotrol	glipizide	Sulfonylurea (Antidiabetic)
Cozaar	losartan	ARB (Angiotensin receptor blocker)
Reglan	metoclopramide	Antiemetic
Nolvadex	tamoxifen	SERM (Selective estrogen receptor modulator)
Micardis	telmisartan	ARB (Angiotensin receptor blocker)
Pepcid	famotidine	H2-receptor antagonist
Buspar	buspirone	Anxiolytic
Duragesic	fentanyl (transdermal)	Opioid analgesic
Ortho-Tri-Cyclen	ethinyl estradiol/norgestimate	Oral contraceptive
Clozaril	clozapine	Atypical antipsychotic
Asacol	mesalamine	Anti-inflammatory (for IBD)
Azmacort	triamcinolone (inhalation)	Corticosteroid (inhalation)

Brand Name	Generic Name	Drug Classification
Aldactone	spironolactone	Diuretic
Lotrel	amlodipine/benazepril	Calcium channel blocker + ACE inhibitor
Zantac	ranitidine	H2-receptor antagonist
Zanaflex	tizanidine	Muscle relaxant
Mevacor	lovastatin	Statin
Proscar	finasteride	5-alpha reductase inhibitor
Remeron	mirtazapine	Antidepressant
Prinzide/Zestoretic	lisinopril/hydrochlorothiazide	ACE inhibitor + Diuretic
Zyban	bupropion (smoking cessation)	Dopamine reuptake inhibitor
Restoril	temazepam	Benzodiazepine (for insomnia)
Tessalon	benzonatate	Antitussive
Betapace	sotalol	Beta-blocker
Cymbalta	duloxetine	SNRI antidepressant
Starlix	nateglinide	Antidiabetic
Lotrisone	clotrimazole/betamethasone	Antifungal + Steroid
Trileptal	oxcarbazepine	Antiepileptic
Aralen	chloroquine	Antimalarial
Toradol	ketorolac	NSAID
Requip	ropinirole	Anti-Parkinson's
Combivent	albuterol/ipratropium	Bronchodilator
Norvir	ritonavir	Antiretroviral
Pamelor	nortriptyline	Tricyclic antidepressant
Vyvanse	lisdexamfetamine	CNS stimulant (for ADHD)
Tegretol	carbamazepine	Antiepileptic
Symbicort	budesonide/formoterol	Corticosteroid + Bronchodilator
Medrol	methylprednisolone	Corticosteroid
Abilify	aripiprazole	Atypical antipsychotic
Exforge	amlodipine/valsartan	CCB + ARB combination
Depakene	valproic acid	Antiepileptic
Nexium	esomeprazole	Proton pump inhibitor
Haldol	haloperidol	Typical antipsychotic
Colace	docusate	Stool softener
Diovan	valsartan	ARB (Angiotensin receptor blocker)
Prezista	darunavir	Antiretroviral
Bactrim, Septra	sulfamethoxazole/trimethoprim	Antibiotic
Xalatan	latanoprost	Prostaglandin (glaucoma treatment)
Sinemet	carbidopa/levodopa	Anti-Parkinson's
Onglyza	saxagliptin	DPP-4 inhibitor (Antidiabetic)

Brand Name	Generic Name	Drug Classification
Femara	letrozole	Aromatase inhibitor (breast cancer)
Atrovent	ipratropium	Anticholinergic bronchodilator
Detrol	tolterodine	Antimuscarinic (overactive bladder)
Phenergan	promethazine	Antiemetic
AndroGel	testosterone (gel)	Testosterone replacement
Prevacid	lansoprazole	Proton pump inhibitor
Methergine	methylergonovine	Uterine contractant
Synthroid	levothyroxine	Thyroid hormone replacement
Vytorin	ezetimibe/simvastatin	Cholesterol-lowering combination
Janumet	sitagliptin/metformin	DPP-4 inhibitor + Biguanide (Antidiabetic)
Invokana	canagliflozin	SGLT2 inhibitor (Antidiabetic)
Motrin	ibuprofen	NSAID
Flomax	tamsulosin	Alpha-1 blocker
Flexeril	cyclobenzaprine	Muscle relaxant
Prograf	tacrolimus	Immunosuppressant
Benicar	olmesartan	ARB (Angiotensin receptor blocker)
Actos	pioglitazone	Thiazolidinedione (Antidiabetic)
Nasonex	mometasone (nasal spray)	Corticosteroid (nasal)
Lyrica	pregabalin	Antiepileptic/Antineuralgic
Aldara	imiquimod	Immune response modifier (topical)
Altace	ramipril	ACE inhibitor
Valtrex	valacyclovir	Antiviral
Effexor XR	venlafaxine	SNRI antidepressant
Avapro	irbesartan	ARB (Angiotensin receptor blocker)
Patanol	olopatadine (eye drops)	Antihistamine (ophthalmic)
Seroquel XR	quetiapine	Atypical antipsychotic
Kaletra	lopinavir/ritonavir	Antiretroviral combination
Zofran	ondansetron	Antiemetic
Zestril, Prinivil	lisinopril	ACE inhibitor
Cogentin	benztropine	Anticholinergic (for Parkinson's)
Humalog	insulin lispro	Rapid-acting insulin
Topamax	topiramate	Antiepileptic
Bystolic	nebivolol	Beta-blocker
Advair Diskus	fluticasone/salmeterol	Corticosteroid + Bronchodilator
Lantus	insulin glargine	Long-acting insulin
Diovan HCT	valsartan/hydrochlorothiazide	ARB + Diuretic combination
Inderal	propranolol	Beta-blocker
Lamictal	lamotrigine	Antiepileptic

Brand Name	Generic Name	Drug Classification
Travatan Z	travoprost (eye drops)	Prostaglandin (glaucoma treatment)
Vesicare	solifenacin	Antimuscarinic (overactive bladder)
Asmanex Twisthaler	mometasone (inhalation)	Corticosteroid (inhalation)
Levitra	vardenafil	Phosphodiesterase-5 inhibitor (Erectile Dysfunction)
Strattera	atomoxetine	Norepinephrine reuptake inhibitor (for ADHD)
Fosamax	alendronate	Bisphosphonate (for osteoporosis)
Celebrex	celecoxib	NSAID (COX-2 inhibitor)
Catapres	clonidine	Alpha-2 agonist (for hypertension)
Lunesta	eszopiclone	Non-benzodiazepine sedative
Crestor	rosuvastatin	Statin (cholesterol-lowering)
Aggrenox	aspirin/dipyridamole	Antiplatelet agent
Lotensin	benazepril	ACE inhibitor
Evista	raloxifene	SERM (Selective Estrogen Receptor Modulator)
Boniva	ibandronate	Bisphosphonate (for osteoporosis)
Dilantin	phenytoin	Antiepileptic
Neurontin	gabapentin	Antiepileptic/Antineuralgic
Ambien CR	zolpidem	Sedative
Exelon	rivastigmine	Cholinesterase inhibitor (for Alzheimer's)
Namenda	memantine	NMDA antagonist (for Alzheimer's)
Januvia	sitagliptin	DPP-4 inhibitor (Antidiabetic)

Pharmacology for Technicians

Patient's Medical History

The medical history of a patient may contain the following details:

- Medications used by the patient, including OTC and nutritional supplements
- Chronic medical conditions
- Acute medical conditions
- Patterns of prescription compliance
- Allergies to items, including drugs and food
- Any interactions that may occur, including drug-drug, drug-food, and so forth".

Understanding a patient's medical history enables the pharmacist to identify any potential risks to the patient. For example, some medical problems may preclude the usage of particular drugs. An allergy to one medicine may signal an allergy to others in the same class. Many drugs are known to interact with each other. Knowing a patient's medication history can help prevent potentially dangerous drug interactions.

OTC Medications and Dietary Supplements

OTC drugs are those that are accessible **"over the counter,"** which means they do not require a prescription. The Federal Food, Drug, and Cosmetic Act requires the FDA to regulate both the sale and manufacture of over-the-counter pharmaceuticals. Certain over-the-counter drugs, such as those containing pseudoephedrine or emergency contraception, require counseling or a signed logbook before being sold by a qualified pharmacy employee due to federal or state laws. Local rules may make a medication available over the counter in one area of the country but only via prescription in another.

Dietary supplements

Dietary supplements, unlike over-the-counter pharmaceuticals, are not FDA-regulated. The Dietary Health and Supplement Act of 1994 defines dietary supplements as any product that meets the following criteria:

- Contains a vitamin, mineral, herb, botanical, and/or amino acid
- Available as a capsule, tablet, powder, or liquid.
- Not meant as the sole source of nutrition.
- Contains the labeling "dietary supplement"

OTC Medications Ingredients

Many over-the-counter medicines contain a combination of different substances, particularly those meant to treat coughs, colds, and the flu. When purchasing over-the-counter pharmaceuticals (or "selling them"), it is critical to double-check the components to ensure that no medications are being replicated. For example, Theraflu and Nyquil both include acetaminophen and dextromethorphan, two drugs that might be harmful if used in excess. Additionally, over-the-counter sleep aids usually include the same chemicals as antihistamines. Migraine recipes commonly contain caffeine, which, if drunk in excess, can produce insomnia and jitteriness. If you are selling medications and see a possible doubling of active components, notify the pharmacist so that he or she can advise the patient.

Chronic Conditions Verses Acute Conditions

Chronic illnesses can develop slowly, over time, and remain persistent. They may go into remission and then reappear. A chronic condition might be moderate, severe, or lethal in nature. Chronic illnesses may necessitate long-term medical care that focuses on symptom alleviation rather than cure. Chronic conditions include heart disease, diabetes, and cancer.

Acute conditions can arise unexpectedly and resolve quickly. Symptoms may be severe. Acute conditions, like chronic ones, can be mild, severe, or even fatal. Acute conditions include strep throat, pneumonia, and gastroenteritis.

Compliance

Compliant patients are conscientious about following their medical providers' advice. Patients take prescribed drugs and undergo essential testing and procedures. Examples of noncompliance are:

- Taking less of the medication than was prescribed
- Stopping medication early
- Taking medication at the wrong time of day
- Using expired medications

Failure to take a prescription as prescribed may result in the medication not working properly or causing undesired side effects. Noncompliance can be caused by a variety of circumstances, including physical concerns, cognitive problems, a fear of adverse effects, and misunderstandings. Pharmacies have implemented mechanisms to improve patient compliance, including as automated refills, sending reminders via phone, text, or email, and notifying doctors of non-compliance.

Medication Allergy

Symptoms of an allergy to a drug include:

- Skin responses include redness and rashes.
- Hives
- Swelling can develop in the face, neck, tongue, or other parts of the body.
- Difficulty breathing, wheezing, or chest tightness

- A rapid or erratic heartbeat

If these symptoms are strong, they could indicate an anaphylactic reaction. Anaphylaxis is a life-threatening condition that requires prompt emergency care. If someone is suspected of experiencing an anaphylactic reaction to any chemical, call 911 right once. Patients may conflate unpleasant effects with allergic reactions. When a patient reports an allergic reaction to a medicine, inquire about the symptoms in order to appropriately identify the reaction.

Food or Medication Allergy History

Some drugs and supplements that may be recommended to a patient include food-based substances. For example, pharmaceutical coatings may contain a variety of incipient components such as lactose, maltodextrin, and other starches, which may cause an allergic reaction in someone who is allergic to those ingredients. Peanut oil is found in a number of prescription lotions as well as the hormone medicine Prometrium. A person with a seafood allergy may need to avoid some omega-3 supplements and shellfish-derived calcium products.Vegan patients will not want to take gelatin capsules, and patients with celiac disease or gluten intolerance should avoid drugs containing gluten fillers. If in doubt, contact the manufacturer.

Drug Interactions

Drug-drug interactions occur when the ingredients of one drug react with the chemicals of another. They may impair the other drug's absorption, neutralize its effect, or enhance its effectiveness. In certain situations, drug manufacturers have taken advantage of this interaction by combining two treatments that are more effective when taken together than alone.

Drug-food interactions occur when specific foods alter the activity of a drug. Some meals may interfere with drug absorption, whilst others may bind to the medication and alter its function. Some prescriptions should be taken with meals, while others are best taken on an empty stomach.

Drug-condition interactions occur when a patient's condition influences how a drug works or when the medication may exacerbate the patient's condition. Certain nasal decongestants, for example, can be problematic for those with high blood pressure, and blood thinners such as aspirin and warfarin should be avoided by people with clotting disorders.

Adverse Drug Reactions

An adverse drug reaction is an undesirable reaction that occurs when a medication is taken in accordance with its recommended dose. Adverse drug reactions might start immediately after taking a medication or develop gradually. Adverse medication effects might be localized or systemic. Serious adverse medication reactions necessitate medical intervention to prevent lasting harm or impairment, and may end in hospitalization or death. There are several possible reactions:

- increased pharmaceutical effects, including intolerance and adverse effects.
- Irregular and unpredictable effects
- Chronic effects

- Delayed effects
- End of treatment effects
- Therapy failure
- Genetic reactions

Polypharmacy

Polypharmacy happens when a patient is taking more medications than are truly required to address their disease. This circumstance is most common among the elderly and persons who are treating various medical diseases, although it can also occur in the general population. One of the most common issues with polypharmacy is the possibility of severe medication interactions. In addition, a variety of pharmacological side effects may develop. Polypharmacy happens when a patient sees many doctors for various diseases, and each doctor is unaware of what the others are prescribing. Pharmacy technicians can prevent polypharmacy by advising pharmacists about medication interactions and multiple prescriptions from various doctors. Pharmacists can assist by consulting with the patient's doctors to ensure that each understands what the other has prescribed and evaluating the prescriptions with the patient and/or caregiver.

Routes of Administration

Medications can be supplied by a variety of methods. Some of the most common include:

- **Orally** or by mouth, such as pills, capsules, elixirs, and suspensions.
- **Nasally**, or by nose, such as nasal sprays or drips
- **Intravenously**, or through the veins
- **Intramuscularly**, or into the muscle
- **Subcutaneous**, or under the skin
- **Epidural**, or infusion into the epidural space
- **Transdermal**, or absorbed through the skin, such as patches and creams
- **Rectally**, or through the anus, such as suppositories and some creams
- **Sublingual**, or under the tongue
- **Inhalation**, or inhaled into the lungs, such as many sprays and nebulized solutions
- **Ocular**, or into the eye, such as many solutions and suspensions
- **Aurally**, or into the ear, such as many solutions and suspensions

Tablet, Capsule, Elixir, and Suspension

The tablet is the most used oral dose type. It may be made of powder that has been tightly crushed into a tablet shape and coated to prevent a bad taste or to postpone medicine delivery. Tablets can also be more complicated, including delayed release mechanisms such as the osmotic release system. Capsules contain pellets, powders, or liquids with a hard or soft gelling agent coating. Many capsules are constructed of gelatin, an animal byproduct, whereas others are made of plant-based polysaccharides. Elixirs are liquid solutions. The active components are dissolved in a liquid carrier. The ingredients in solutions do not need to be shaken together. A suspension is made up of drugs suspended in a liquid carrier. Before being administered to the patient, some suspensions must be mixed with distilled water first. Suspensions must be shaken before use, as the contents may settle.

IV Admixture

IV admixture is a sort of compounding in which a medicine is added to a 50 mL or larger container of fluid that will be delivered intravenously. Proper IV mixing necessitates skill and experience, as it is critical to administer the correct amount of medication to the patient with no margin for error. Successful IV admixture requires knowledge of good aseptic technique. Failure to use adequate method may result in the patient being overdosed or underdosed, as well as the introduction of hazardous microorganisms or other toxins into the patient's system.

Drawing a Drug from an Ampule

When utilizing a medication stored in an ampule, particular precautions must be taken to avoid injury when opening the ampule and to prevent particles such as paint chips and glass from entering the medicine.

1. To remove medication from the tip, flick or tap the top of the ampule.

2. Wipe the top of the ampule with an alcohol swab.

3. Wrap the tip in gauze and rapidly snap it off, away from your body and face.

4. Using a syringe fitted with a filter needle, remove the exact amount of medication while keeping the needle away from the ampule's edges.

5. Ampule may be tipped slightly in order to withdraw all the medication.

6. Before injecting the drug, the filter needle must be removed and a sterile normal needle inserted.

7. Place the filter needle and both components of the ampule in the sharps container.

Pharmacokinetics

Pharmacokinetics refers to the mechanism by which the body metabolizes medications. Understanding the pharmacokinetics of a medicine is crucial for determining its rate of metabolization and elimination by the body. Pharmacokinetics is divided into four stages: **absorption, distribution, metabolism**, and **elimination**. It's challenging to anticipate how a medicine will be absorbed in a certain patient due to individual factors influencing the rate. Some of the factors that influence the rate of metabolism include:

- Patient's age
- Recent food, drink or alcohol consumption
- The effect of other medications that have been taken

"Half-Life"

The body will metabolize and remove a portion of the substance during the course of a given time unit. During each half-life period, half of the drug contained in the blood is digested and removed. Although drugs are in the same class, the effects of one may persist longer than those of another. This is due in part to the medication's half-life. A medication with a half-life of 14 hours eliminates half of its blood concentration in every 14-hour increment, whereas a medication with a half-life of 5 hours eliminates half its blood concentration in each 5-hour increment. This means that the medicine with a 5-hour half-life will leave the body significantly faster.

The medication's half-life dictates the dosing rate. The medicine with a 5-hour half-life may need to be dosed twice daily, but the 14-hour half-life medication just has to be dosed once daily.

Zero Order Kinetics

Zero order kinetics states that your body processes a drug at a constant rate, regardless of its concentration in your bloodstream. The body normally processes alcohol in a zero-kinetic mode.For instance, if your body can handle 1 ounce of alcohol each hour, but you consume 3 ounces in an hour, your body will still process it at the same pace. After one hour, your body will have processed one ounce of alcohol, two hours, the second ounce of alcohol, and three hours, the third ounce. If you do not consume any additional alcohol after those three ounces, you will no longer have alcohol in your system.

Age of Person Affect Response of Medication

The extremely young and the very old frequently have distinct reactions to drugs. They may respond to the strength differently than expected, develop unique side effects, or a dose that appears correct when calculated by weight may be an overdose. Many drugs have not been approved by the FDA for use in children, but are "used off label." Many drugs have not been investigated in pediatric or geriatric populations, thus unexpected reactions may occur. If a physician prescribes a medicine that is not approved for use in either of these categories, contact the pharmacist, who will use professional judgment to determine whether to distribute the medication or notify the physician.

Abbreviations

When a Medication Should Be Taken

Abbreviation	Meaning
ac	before meals
bid	twice daily
hs	at bedtime
pc	after meals
prn	as needed
q4h/q4	every 4 hours
qd	daily
qid	four times daily
qod	every other day
tid	three times daily

Drug Dosage

Abbreviation	Meaning
cap	capsule
gtt	drop
I, ii, iii, iv	1, 2, 3, 4 (Roman numerals are often used to identify quantities on prescriptions)
mcg/μg	microgram (μg is not being used as much because when written out, it is often mistaken for mg. If unsure, confirm dose with prescriber)
mg	milligram
mL	milliliter
ss	one-half
tab	tablet
tbsp.	tablespoon (15 ml)
tsp.	teaspoon (4 ml)

Route of Administration

Abbreviation	Meaning
ad	right ear
as	left ear
au	both ears
c	with
od	right eye
os	left eye
ou	both eyes
po	by mouth
sl	sublingual
top	topically

Sample Sigs

Sigs	Understandable dosing instructions
i tab po bid prn	Take one tablet by mouth twice daily as needed
ii gtts au tid	Instill two drops in both ears three times daily
i–ii tabs q4–6h prn pain	Take one to two tablets every four to six hours as needed for pain
apply top qd	Apply topically once daily
i–ii tsp po tid ac	Take one to two teaspoons by mouth three times daily before meals
5–10 ml po q8h prn cough	Take 5–10 ml by mouth every eight hours as needed for cough. (Alternatively, take 1 to 2 teaspoons by mouth every eight hours as needed for cough)
Inj 3 units sq pc	Inject 3 units subcutaneously after meals
i gtt os q2	Instill one drop in the left eye every two hours
ii cap po qhs	Take two capsules by mouth every night at bedtime
I tab qam, may repeat xl prn	Take one tablet every morning. May repeat once

Drug Abbreviation

Many drugs are designated using common acronyms. Here are some of the most common:

Common Abbreviation	Medication
APAP	acetaminophen
ASA	aspirin
Fe	iron
HCTZ	hydrochlorothiazide
INH	isoniazid
MgSO4	magnesium sulfate
MOM	milk of magnesia
MVI	multivitamin
NS	normal saline
NTG	nitroglycerin
PCN	penicillin
PNV	prenatal vitamins
SMZ/TMP	sulfamethoxazole/trimethoprim
TAC	triamcinolone
TCN	tetracycline

Body Systems

The Nervous System

The nervous system is actually divided into two parts: the central nervous system (CNS) and the peripheral nervous system (PNS). The central nervous system consists of two major organs: the spinal cord and the brain. The rest of the nerves in the body make up the PNS. The nervous system's function is to send impulses from the nerves to the brain and vice versa. The brain is divided into three sections: the forebrain, which stores an individual's unique information; the midbrain, which controls signals that pass via the spinal cord; and the hindbrain, which coordinates movement. The majority of nervous system activity is carried out by neurons, which are highly specialized in terms of function and transport messages via a very complex chemical process.

The Immune System

The immune system fights disease within the body, keeping it healthy and free of infection. The immune system consists of five major components: the thymus, spleen, lymphatic system, white blood cells, and bone marrow. The immune system acts in three distinct ways.

- It works to prevent infections from ever entering the body.
- If a foreign body enters the body, the immune system attempts to recognize and destroy it.
- If bacteria or viruses enter the body and reproduce, the immune system fights the infection and eliminates it.

In some cases, the immune system may malfunction and misinterpret the body's own system for external contaminants, resulting in an immunological response. These are autoimmune diseases like lupus, rheumatoid arthritis, and multiple sclerosis.

The Digestive System

The digestive system transforms food into energy for the rest of the body and eliminates waste. The digestive system's main organs are the mouth, esophagus, stomach, liver, gallbladder, pancreas, small and large intestines, and rectum. When food is digested, it is broken down in the mouth by chewing and enzymes in saliva. The meal passes via the esophagus and into the stomach, where it is further broken down by gastric acid. It next enters the small intestine, where bile, which is produced by the liver and stored in the gall bladder, interacts with digestive enzymes produced by the pancreas and intestines to further digest the food. Some nutrients are also absorbed in the small intestine. Water and electrolytes are absorbed from the food as it passes through the large intestine. The leftover waste remains in the rectum until evacuated by the anus.

The Circulatory System

The circulatory system consists mostly of veins, arteries, blood cells, and the heart. Oxygenated blood enters the heart and exits through the left ventricle into the aorta, the largest artery. Blood circulates through the body's arteries. Once the oxygen is used up, the blood returns to the heart via the veins, passing through the lungs to remove carbon dioxide. Blood is oxygenated in the lungs before returning to the heart. The heart is a sophisticated organ made up of cardiac muscle, a type of striated involuntary muscle.

The Reproductive System

The male reproductive system is mostly composed of the penis, scrotum, and testes. The testes, often known as testicles, make testosterone and sperm. The scrotum protects the testicles and regulates the temperature necessary for sperm production. When a man ejaculates, semen (a protective fluid containing sperm) is released from the testes and travels down the vas deferens to the urethra, which passes through the center of the prostate gland before exiting through the penis. The female reproductive system consists of the ovaries, fallopian tubes, uterus, cervix, and vagina. About once a month, one of the ovaries develops an egg, which travels down the fallopian tube to the uterus. If the egg is not fertilized, the lining that grew to prepare for the fertilized egg is eliminated during menstruation. If sperm fertilizes the egg, it will implant in the uterus. Over the next 40 weeks, it will develop into a baby. The baby is born during labor, which requires passage via the cervix and vagina.

The Endocrine System

The endocrine system secretes hormones that regulate practically every other organ and system in the body. The endocrine system influences mood, development, metabolism, growth, tissue function, and various other activities. The endocrine system consists of the hypothalamus, pituitary gland, pineal gland, thyroid and parathyroid glands, and adrenal gland. The heart, kidneys, stomach, pancreas, intestines, testes in men, and ovaries in women are all auxiliary organs that generate hormones and are part of the endocrine system. The glands secrete hormones, which travel throughout the body to cells with receptors that can absorb the hormone and exchange chemical information.

The Lymphatic System

The lymphatic system works with the circulatory and immune systems to keep the body healthy and prevent illness. The lymphatic system includes the tonsils, adenoids, thymus, spleen, lymph nodes, and lymph, a clear fluid made up of white blood cells and a protective component called chyle. Lymph moves through a complex system of lymph nodes, ducts, and veins. Lymph nodes filter the lymph as it passes through. When bacteria or other infectious agents are identified, the nodes grow and create more white blood cells to help the immune system fight the infection.

The Muscular System

The muscular system is divided into three categories of muscles: skeletal, cardiac, and smooth (or visceral). Muscle fibers expand and contract, allowing movement throughout the body. The human body has approximately 650 different muscles, each with a specific function.

- **Skeletal muscles** are striated, with bands of light and dark layers. They are attached to the skeleton by tendons and are the muscles that are consciously controlled and exercised.
- **Cardiac muscle** is likewise striated, although its action is not under conscious control. The heart muscle helps to maintain blood circulating through the circulatory system. During hard exercise, the heart can boost its output by up to five times in order to keep oxygenated blood flowing to the muscles.
- The **smooth or visceral muscles** are found throughout the systems of the body and work to keep the blood vessels and other organs working properly. These muscles are not under conscious control.

The Skeletal System

The skeletal system provides stability and support for your body. The skull, ribs, and pelvis are bone structures that protect the body's most important organs, such as the brain, heart, and lungs. Tendons connect muscles and bones, allowing for movement. The skeletal system's major bone structures include the skull, spine, ribs, humerus, radius and ulna, pelvis, femur, fibula, and tibia. The bones are formed of several layers. A dense outer layer shields a flexible, spongy layer. The bone marrow, which runs through the center of many bones in the skeleton, creates new blood cells and aids in the immune system's proper function.

The Urinary System

The urinary system's core consists of the kidneys, ureters, bladder, and urethra. The kidney's principal function is to filter waste from the blood and produce urine. Urine travels from the kidneys to the ureters and bladder before exiting through the urethra. Nerves in the bladder give signals to the brain when it is full and peeing is required to empty it. Sphincter muscles restrict the bladder's opening, allowing the body to hold urine without releasing it.

Common Chronic Conditions

Type 2 Diabetes

The risk factors for type 2 diabetes include:

- Excess weight
- Hypertension
- Prediabetes or reduced glucose tolerance.
- A sedentary lifestyle
- Insulin resistance
- Genetics
- Ethnic background (diabetes is more common in those of Hispanic, African, Native American, and Asian descent)
- Increased age
- History of gestational diabetes
- Polycystic ovary syndrome

Patients with these risk factors may be able to halt the progression of Type 2 diabetes by losing weight and modifying their lifestyle. Even after a diagnosis, lifestyle adjustments and weight loss can help prevent diabetes from worsening and allow the patient to manage it without medication. Counseling can assist patients in adopting better habits.

Rosiglitazone, Metformin, Glargine, and Detemir

Diabetes treatments include rosiglitazone, metformin, glargine, and detemir. Diabetes is a chronic condition in which the body is unable to regulate blood sugar levels due to insufficient insulin synthesis or insulin resistance. Diabetes is classified into two types: Type 1 and Type 2. **Type 1** diabetes usually occurs in early childhood. **Type 2** diabetes appears later in life and is commonly connected with poor eating and exercise habits, although there is also likely to be a hereditary component. While diabetes rarely causes symptoms in everyday life, symptoms might emerge when blood sugar levels become abnormally high or low. Some of the symptoms include thirst or hunger, fatigue, blurred vision, tingling in the feet, and frequent urination.

Checking Blood Sugar

Patients with diabetes should test their blood sugar on a regular basis to ensure that it is within control. Fluctuating blood sugar levels suggest that a patient's diabetes is not under control. Most blood glucose monitors work in a similar fashion. The patient pricks his or her finger with a lancet and applies a drop of blood to a test strip. The testing strip is then placed in the meter, which monitors blood sugar levels. Most modern machines require only a small amount of blood to acquire an accurate reading and return the result in seconds. Advanced meters can store readings over time, allowing doctors to track blood sugar levels.

Heart Disease

The risk factors for heart disease are:

- Being male, but a woman's risk increases after menopause.
- Increased age
- Genetics
- Ethnicity (heart disease is more common in those of African, Native American, or Hispanic descent)
- Smoking
- High LDL cholesterol
- High blood pressure
- A sedentary lifestyle
- Poorly controlled diabetes
- High levels of stress and anger
- High C-reactive protein

Patients cannot change their race, age, or family history, but they can undertake a number of lifestyle changes to reduce their risk of cardiovascular disease. Quitting smoking, eating a low-saturated fat and high fiber diet, and practicing better stress management strategies can all help reduce your risk of developing heart disease.

High Cholesterol

The risk factors for high cholesterol include:

- Gender (a woman's LDL level increases following menopause)
- A diet high in saturated fat and cholesterol
- Increased age
- Excess weight
- A sedentary lifestyle

While some people develop high cholesterol owing to genetics, many more do so as a result of their lifestyle choices. High cholesterol can be reduced by making significant lifestyle changes, such as increasing exercise and eating low-saturated-fat meals with whole grains and fresh fruit and vegetables. When LDLs are too high and HDLs are too low, boosting the LDL/HDL ratio can help. Eating fatty fish, which are high in omega-3s, as well as olive oil, a monounsaturated fat, and getting plenty of exercise can help you boost your LDL to HDL ratio.

Simvastatin, pravastatin, atorvastatin, and rosuvastatin

Simvastatin, pravastatin, atorvastatin, and rosuvastatin are all medications used to treat high cholesterol. High cholesterol rarely produces symptoms, but it does cause fatty deposits to develop in the blood vessels. Over time, these deposits impede the flow of blood through the veins. When the blood supply to the heart is decreased, a heart attack can occur. When the blood supply to the brain is limited, a stroke may occur. While high cholesterol is hereditary, a healthy diet and regular exercise can help prevent it. The total cholesterol has two components: HDL (good cholesterol) and LDL (bad cholesterol).Lowering total cholesterol is beneficial, but keeping a high HDL-to-LDL ratio is even more important.

Statin Medications

Statins are a class of medications used to treat high cholesterol. While using this medication, you should avoid drinking grapefruit juice or eating grapefruit in large amounts. Grapefruit juice stops your body from adequately breaking down medicines, allowing the statin to build in your system. This raises the risk of serious adverse effects like muscle or liver damage.

The pharmacist should teach the patient how to avoid grapefruit juice while taking statins. Increasing medicine dosage may appear beneficial, but excessive amounts might be difficult for the liver to process. Muscle injury is indicated by sudden muscle discomfort, which should be treated by a medical practitioner immediately.

Rhabdomyolysis

Rhabdomyolysis is a serious, and occasionally fatal, adverse effect of statin medications. Under these conditions, skeletal muscle tissue degrades and is destroyed rapidly. All statin patients should be educated on the need of obtaining prescribed blood tests and reporting any symptoms of muscle pain or fatigue to their doctors immediately. Failure to recognize and treat rhabdomyolysis might result in mortality. While statins are the most well-known, additional pharmaceuticals linked to rhabdomyolysis include Parkinson's disease therapies, anesthetics, colchicine, and several HIV meds.

High Blood Pressure

High blood pressure is related to the following risk factors:

- Increased age
- Ethnicity (African Americans are more likely to develop high blood pressure)
- Genetics
- Excess weight
- A sedentary lifestyle
- Tobacco use
- Excess dietary sodium
- Insufficient dietary potassium
- Excess use of alcohol
- High stress levels

- Other chronic illnesses include diabetes, high cholesterol, renal disease, and sleep apnea.

High blood pressure is a risk factor for major illnesses like heart disease and stroke, so it's vital to keep it under control. Patients can lower their blood pressure by stopping smoking, losing weight, eating a nutritious diet, and exercising regularly.

Metoprolol, Amlodipine, Valsartan, and Lisinopril

Metoprolol, amlodipine, valsartan, and lisinopril are all drugs used to treat hypertension. High blood pressure is a frequent and hazardous condition that affects multiple body systems. It is usually asymptomatic, however some people have dizziness or headaches. Untreated high blood pressure leads to coronary artery disease, heart failure, kidney failure, and stroke. Blood pressure is measured in two parts: systolic (highest) and diastolic (lowest). Adults with normal blood pressure have systolic pressures less than 120 mmHg and diastolic pressures less than 80 mmHg. High blood pressure develops in three stages:

- **Prehypertension** (systolic of 120 – 139 and diastolic of 80– 89)
- **Stage 1** (systolic of 150 – 159 and diastolic of 90 – 99)
- **Stage 2** (systolic of 160 or higher and diastolic of 100 or higher)

Antihypertensive Medications

The following antihypertensive medications have common dose ranges, formulations, and routes of administration:

1. **Hydrochlorothiazide** – The suggested HCTZ dosage is 25 mg to 100 mg per day. It can be taken in a single dose or divided throughout the day. HCTZ is available as oral capsules, tablets, and solutions.
2. **Atenolol** – Depending on the circumstances, atenolol is often dosed at 50 mg to 100 mg daily, with a maximum of 200 mg daily. Atenolol is offered as oral pills and intravenous injections.
3. **Amlodipine** – Amlodipine doses range from 2.5 mg to 10 mg daily. It's accessible as an oral tablet.
4. **Benazepril** – The normal daily dose of benazepril is between 5 mg to 80 mg. Benazepril is available as an oral tablet.
5. **Losartan** – Losartan is typically dosed at 25 to 100 mg per day, it may be taken in a single daily dose or divided into two doses. It is available as an oral tablet.

ACE Inhibitors

Angiotensin converting enzyme (ACE) inhibitors are used to treat hypertension and congestive heart failure. As the name implies, the medication inhibits the release of the angiotensin converting enzyme. This decreases blood volume and tension in the arteries, lowering blood pressure.

The most common ACE inhibitors are:

- Lisinopril
- Enalapril

- Captopril
- Ramipril

ACE inhibitors frequently cause the following negative effects:

- Cough
- Low blood pressure
- Dizziness
- Fatigue
- Headache
- Hyperkalemia

The most common ACE inhibitor-related side effect is chronic dry cough. While the cough is not dangerous, it can be irritating, and some people may require a different medication to manage their hypertension.

Calcium Channel Blockers

Calcium channel blockers stop calcium from passing through calcium channels. This inhibits the contraction of vascular smooth muscle, causing blood vessel dilation. This lowers blood pressure and makes the heart work less. These medications are used to treat hypertension, regulate the heart rate, and prevent angina.

Common calcium channel blockers include:

- Amlodipine
- Felodipine
- Nifedipine
- Verapamil
- Diltiazem

Side effects of calcium channel blockers include:

- Dizziness
- Flushing
- Headache
- Edema
- Tachycardia
- Bradycardia
- Constipation

When used with other hypertensive medications, CCB toxicity is possible. Certain combinations, such as verapamil and beta blockers, may cause severe bradycardia.

Vasodilators

Vasodilators dilate blood arteries, allowing blood to flow more freely. This minimizes the amount of work necessary for the heart to pump blood throughout the body. Vasodilators are prescribed to manage excessive blood pressure, angina, and heart failure. Nitroglycerin, the most commonly used vasodilator, is available in a variety of forms, including sublingual pills, extended release capsules, and transdermal patches/creams. Other vasodilators that may be used include minoxidil and alprostadil, albeit these medicines are also promoted in ways that exploit their negative effects (for example, minoxidil for hair growth).

Common adverse effects related with vasodilators are:

- Lightheadedness
- Dizziness
- Low blood pressure
- Flushing

Vasodilators should not be taken with some medications, particularly those used to treat erectile dysfunction. This can result in a fatal drop in blood pressure.

Nitroglycerin

Nitroglycerin is a vasodilator that is widely prescribed to alleviate angina, or chest pain. To avoid recurrent angina, prolonged release nitroglycerin capsules are taken daily, with sublingual tablets or sprays used on occasion. Nitroglycerin should not be taken with the erectile dysfunction medicines sildenafil, tadalafil, or vardenafil. These medicines enhance the effects of nitroglycerin and can cause permanent hypotension, which can be fatal. If this combination occurs accidently, seek emergency medical help right once. Symptoms of hypotension include dizziness, fainting, and cold, clammy skin.

Alpha-Agonist Hypotensive Agents

Alpha-agonist hypotensive medicines, often known as alpha-blockers, keep small blood vessels open by relaxing specific muscle groups. Norepinephrine, the hormone that tightens muscles in the walls of small blood arteries, is blocked, enabling the vessels to remain open and relaxed, decreasing blood pressure. These medications are prescribed to treat both high blood pressure and benign prostatic hyperplasia.

Examples of alpha agonist hypotensive drugs are:

- Doxazosin
- Prazosin
- Tamsulosin
- Alfuzosin

Some typical adverse effects connected with alpha-blockers are:

- Low blood pressure
- Dizziness

- Headache
- Pounding heartbeat
- Weakness
- Nausea
- Weight gain
- Decreases in LDL cholesterol

Diuretics

Diuretics are generally used to treat high blood pressure and have a number of common side effects, including:

Frequent urination — Diuretics assist the body shed excess water through urination. As a result, the drug is frequently administered in the morning to avoid disrupting sleep.

Abnormalities in electrolytes such as potassium or sodium — Patients should have regular blood tests as directed by their doctor to detect these irregularities.

Fatigue or weakness —This effect should lessen as the patient becomes used to the medication.

Dizziness and lightheadedness — Postural hypotension (a sudden drop in blood pressure when getting up quickly) is a common side effect when taking diuretics.

Dehydration — If the dose is too high, the patient may show signs of dehydration.

Loop Diuretics

Loop diuretics work by directly targeting the kidney's Henle loop. The medications inhibit the absorption of salt and chloride. This prevents urine concentration, which leads to greater production. The end result is a decrease in blood volume, which lowers blood pressure and minimizes swelling.

Loop diuretics contain:

- Furosemide
- Torsemide
- Bumetanide

Common side effects of loop diuretics include:

- Low levels of other electrolytes such as potassium and magnesium (potassium and magnesium replacements are commonly administered in conjunction with loop diuretics)
- Dehydration
- Dizziness
- Syncope
- Postural hypotension
- Hyperuricemia

Tinnitus and vertigo when taking loop diuretics may suggest a serious but uncommon side effect known as ototoxicity, which can cause deafness.

Warfarin

Warfarin is a powerful blood thinner. When taking warfarin, patients should exercise caution when taking other drugs to avoid excessive thinning, which can be hazardous. Many painkillers thin the blood or enhance the action of warfarin. Some of these medications are:

- Aspirin
- Acetaminophen
- Ibuprofen
- Naproxen
- Celecoxib
- Diclofenac
- Indomethacin
- Piroxicam

Patients on warfarin should consult with their doctor or pharmacist before beginning any new medication or making dietary changes to ensure its safety. Prolonged bleeding and large bruises from modest traumas are signs of extremely thin blood.

Tachycardia, Bradycardia, and Arrhythmia

Tachycardia is a heartbeat that is quicker than the normal resting pace. This amount changes greatly depending on the person's age and level of fitness. Tachycardia, depending on the rate and quality of the beat, can be dangerous or indicate a serious health concern. Bradycardia is a slow heartbeat. Bradycardia in adults is characterized as a heart rate of fewer than 60 beats per minute. The patient is usually asymptomatic until his or her heart rate drops below 50 beats per minute. A low heart rate could indicate or induce cardiac arrest. Arrhythmia, also known as cardiac dysrhythmia, is defined as any abnormal heartbeat, including tachycardia, bradycardia, and irregular pulse. Some arrhythmias are harmless, but others can indicate a serious condition that requires rapid medical attention.

Depression

Depression is a hazardous condition that, if not treated, can lead to the patient harming themselves or dying by suicide. Depression treatment has a two-pronged approach. Medicine is effective because it regulates serotonin, norepinephrine, and dopamine levels in the brain; however, combining medicine with treatment and counseling increases the patient's capacity to cope with daily tasks. Medication alleviates the chemical imbalances in the brain that cause depression. Talk therapy helps the patient eliminate negative and discouraging thoughts and replace them with positive self-talk and behaviors.

Escitalopram, Venlafaxine, Bupropion, and Sertraline

Escitalopram, venlafaxine, bupropion, and sertraline are all drugs used to treat depression, which is a mood disorder marked by intense feelings of sadness, anger, loss, and frustration.

The exact process of depression is unknown, however most research assume it is a combination of inherited and environmental factors. Depression can afflict everyone, regardless of age, race, gender, or socioeconomic status.

Some frequent symptoms of depression are:

- Difficulty concentrating
- Loss of enthusiasm for formerly enjoyable activity.
- Fatigue
- A feeling of worthlessness or hopelessness.
- Thoughts of suicide
- Difficulty sleeping

Antidepressants are commonly used in conjunction with counseling or mental therapy to treat depression.

Antidepressants

The antidepressants listed below have common dose ranges, formulations, and routes of administration:

1. Amitriptyline – Amitriptyline can be started at a low dose of 10 mg and increased to 300 mg per day. It can be taken as a single dose or in two to three doses per day. Amitriptyline is available in both oral pills and intramuscular injections.
2. Bupropion – The typical adult dose of bupropion is 150 mg to 300 mg per day in divided doses or as a single extended-release tablet. The maximum daily dose is 450 mg per day. Bupropion comes in both regular and extended-release oral tablets.
3. Citalopram – Citalopram is administered in doses ranging from 20 to 40 mg per day. Dosages more than 40 mg per day are not recommended. Citalopram is available as oral pills and a solution.
4. Mirtazapine – Mirtazapine is commonly used at doses ranging from 15 mg to 45 mg per day. Mirtazapine is available as both oral tablets and disintegrating oral tablets.

MAOI

MAOI stands for monoamine oxidase inhibitor. These medications are intended to treat depression. While these were the first types of antidepressants developed, the adverse effect profile and potential for hazardous interactions are so severe that they are currently only used to treat depression that has not responded to other therapy options. Some MAOIs are phenelzine (brand name Nardil), selegiline (brand name Emsam), and tranylcypromine (brand name Parnate). MAOIs can cause a number of side effects, including serotonin syndrome, which happens when a patient's serotonin levels rise dangerously. The symptoms of serotonin syndrome are similar to those of heart attack. Many medications and foods may have substantial side effects when used with MAOIs. Tyramine-containing foods, such as wine, cheese, some meats, and pickled foods, may raise blood pressure when used with MAOIs.

Antipsychotics

The category of atypical antipsychotic medicines includes:

- Aripiprazole
- Clozapine
- Olanzapine
- Quetiapine
- Risperidone
- Ziprasidone

These medications are often used to treat mental illnesses like schizophrenia and bipolar disorder. Other applications include the treatment of anxiety disorders and obsessive-compulsive disorder. The side effects of this class of medications vary. The most prevalent and dangerous side effect is the risk of developing tardive dyskinesia, a disorder marked by repeated, involuntary movements such as foot twisting, mouth smacking, and eye blinking.

Other possible adverse effects are:

- Dystonia
- Reduction in sexual interest
- Abnormal menstrual cycles
- Enlargement of the breasts
- Increased risk of diabetes
- Weight gain

Gastroesophageal Reflux Disease (GERD)

Esomeprazole, Omeprazole, Lansoprazole, and Pantoprazole

Esomeprazole, omeprazole, lansoprazole, and pantoprazole are all medicines used to treat gastroesophageal reflux disease (GERD). In this condition, the lower esophageal sphincter is weak and does not seal properly, allowing stomach contents to back up into the esophagus and create irritation. The most common symptoms of GERD include heartburn, coughing, nausea, difficulty swallowing, and a hoarse voice. A range of factors may contribute to or exacerbate GERD. Obesity, pregnancy, overconsumption of acidic foods, a hiatal hernia, and smoking are just a few instances. In addition to taking medications, persons with GERD can help control their symptoms by avoiding triggering foods, losing weight (if obesity is a contributing factor), eating less at meals, and avoiding lying down immediately after eating.

Asthma

Nebulizer

A nebulizer is a device that aerosolizes liquid medications, allowing patients to easily inhale them. It is often used to treat asthma and pneumonia. Some inhaler medicines come pre-mixed (for example, 0.083% albuterol), whereas others may require the patient to mix them. The nebulizer consists of numerous components: the main machine, the filter, tubing, a holding chamber, and the mouthpiece or mask. To ensure that the machine runs well, each component must be cleaned on a regular basis. Filters, in particular, require regular cleaning or replacement.

Montelukast, Albuterol, Fluticasone, and Budesonide

Asthma is treated with budesonide, fluticasone, albuterol, and montelukast. Asthma causes swelling in the lungs' passages, making breathing difficult and producing symptoms such as wheezing, coughing, chest tightness, and shortness of breath. Asthma is a severe condition that necessitates quick treatment. Untreated asthma can be lethal. Environmental allergies, certain medicines, stress, tobacco use, and respiratory infections are all possible factors for asthma. To stop an asthma attack, a long-acting control therapy (inhaled corticosteroids like fluticasone or leukotriene inhibitors like montelukast) is typically combined with a fast-acting medication like albuterol or ipratropium. To manage asthma, it is necessary to identify and avoid triggers, create an asthma strategy, monitor breathing with a peak flow meter, and adhere to emergency measures.

HIV

HIV is the virus that causes AIDS, a devastating disease in which the immune system is ravaged. Despite major breakthroughs in HIV treatment, there is still no known cure. HIV is transmitted by contact with body fluids.

The most common modes of transmission are:
- Unprotected sexual contact with an infected person
- Sharing needles with an infected person

Children born to infected mothers have a possibility of developing the disease. In the healthcare industry, contact with an infected person's blood or bodily fluids raises the risk of transmission. Medical professionals can protect themselves by using personal protective equipment like gloves and masks, following stringent infection control protocols, and being cautious near needles used to provide injections to patients.

Hepatitis B

Hepatitis B is a viral infection that injures the liver and produces inflammation. It can eventually lead to liver failure and death. Hepatitis B is transmitted through contact with bodily fluids, including
- Unprotected sexual contact
- Tattoos performed with shared instruments
- Sharing needles and other paraphernalia used to inject drugs
- Sharing personal goods, such as razors and toothbrushes.
- Childbirth

If you become exposed to blood or other bodily fluids while working, notify your infection control team right once. Healthcare professionals are considered high-risk, therefore you should receive a hepatitis B vaccine to avoid contracting the disease.

Commonly Prescribed Medications

Antibiotics

The antibiotics listed below have the following usual dose range, dosing forms, and administration methods:

1. Amoxicillin — Amoxicillin is often given at a dose of 250 mg to 500 mg every 8 hours, or 500 mg to 875 mg every 12 hours. Amoxicillin comes in three forms: chewable pills, capsules, and powder for suspension.

2. Penicillin VK — The normal penicillin VK dose is 125 mg to 500 mg every 6 to 8 hours. Penicillin VK is available as oral tablets and powder for suspension.

3. Cephalexin — Cephalexin is commonly used in doses of 250 mg every 6 hours or 500 mg every 12 hours. Cephalexin is available in both oral capsules and powder for suspension.

4. Cefuroxime — Cefuroxime dosages typically vary between 250 mg and 500 mg per 12 hours. It comes in both tablet and powder forms for oral suspension.

5. Azithromycin — Azithromycin can be administered as a single dose of 1000 mg, three daily doses of 500 mg, or one daily dose of 500 mg followed by four daily doses of 250 mg. It is available as oral tablets and powder for oral suspension.

Amoxicillin, Penicillin, Clarithromycin, Tetracycline, and Cephalexin

All of these medications are antibiotics. They cure bacterial diseases. Antibiotics eliminate infections from the body in one of two ways. Some antibiotics, such as penicillin, kill bacteria. Others stop bacteria from developing. Antibiotics are not effective against viral infections. A doctor may test a culture to determine which strain of bacteria is causing the infection, as some bacteria are more vulnerable to certain antibiotic classes. Antibiotic abuse has become a major problem in the United States, with multiple cases of **"superbugs"**—bacteria resistant to all but the most powerful antibiotics.

Controlled Substances

The restricted pharmaceuticals listed below have the following normal dose ranges, dosage forms, and administration methods:

1. Hydrocodone/acetaminophen — The hydrocodone element is available in quantities ranging from 2.5 mg to 10 mg, while the acetaminophen portion ranges from 325 mg to 650 mg. Doses are often one or two pills given at different times throughout the day, depending on the severity of the pain. The maximum daily dose of acetaminophen should not exceed 4000 mg. This medication is available in a range of dosages, including oral pills and an oral solution.

2. Lorazepam — Lorazepam is often administered as needed, up to 6 mg per day in divided doses. Lorazepam is offered as oral pills and injectable solutions.

3. Methylphenidate — Methylphenidate can be taken up to 72 mg per day (under the brand name Concerta). Immediate release tablets can be taken once or twice a day, whereas extended release pills are used once a day. Methylphenidate is available in oral and extended-release pills.

Oral Contraceptives

Oral contraceptives cause a variety of side effects, some of which are significant. Birth control pills increase the risk of potentially fatal blood clots, particularly in women over 35 and those who smoke. Common and less severe side effects include the following:

- Nausea
- Weight gain
- Spotting between periods
- Changes in mood
- Lighter periods
- Aching or swollen breasts

Severe side effects requiring immediate emergency attention include:

- Chest pain
- Blurred vision
- Stomach pain
- Severe headaches

Yasmin, Ortho Tri-Cyclen, Trinessa, Sprintec, and Ovcon

Yasmin, Ortho Tri-Cyclen, TriNessa, Sprintec, and Ovcon are all oral contraceptives, also known as birth control pills or "the pill." Women use them on a daily basis to avoid conception. Oral contraceptives are used in a variety of ways to prevent pregnancy. Oral contraceptives contain estrogen and/or progestin. Progestin-only oral contraceptives include Micronor and Ovrette, popularly known as the "minipill" By delivering a steady supply of these hormones, the hormones that cause eggs to mature and exit the ovary are suppressed. Furthermore, the hormones prevent the endometrium from growing enough to accommodate a fertilized egg. Progestins create a mucus barrier, preventing sperm from fertilizing the egg. It is also thought that progestins modify the fallopian tubes, making it difficult for eggs to pass through them.

Birth Control

Antibiotics are known to reduce or undermine the effectiveness of hormonal birth control. This means that if a woman utilizes oral contraception (or other hormonal methods such as NuvaRing), she may conceive while taking antibiotics. Pharmacists should notify women on antibiotics about the possibility of obtaining birth control from another drugstore or source. To avert an unintended pregnancy, a barrier technique, such as condoms, must be used during antibiotic therapy and for at least two weeks afterward. Anti-fungal drugs, some anti-seizure pharmaceuticals, certain HIV medications, and herbal preparations like St. John's Wort may all have an effect on birth control.

Antihistamines

Although many antihistamines are available over the counter, they can have a number of undesirable side effects. Side effects include the following:

- Drowsiness is a typical side effect, and many antihistamines, including diphenhydramine, are sold as sleep aids under a variety of brand names. Antihistamines should not be used when attention is essential, especially before driving.
- Headaches
- Increased blood pressure
- Stomach upset

Dry mouth and decreased urine (the anticholinergic effect of antihistamines, which helps to dry up a stuffy nose, can also cause drying in other regions of the body).

Potential Side Effects of Chemotherapy

Although chemotherapy is widely used to treat cancer, it is also known to have major adverse effects. To mitigate the side effects of chemotherapy, medications are frequently administered. Some common side effects are:

- Constipation or diarrhea (laxatives or anti-diarrhea drugs like loperamide are frequently recommended along with chemotherapy).
- Fatigue
- Hair Loss
- Weakened immune system leading to infection
- Anemia (IV medicines to promote red blood cell growth, such as darbepoetin alfa, may be administered)
- Loss of appetite (drugs like dronabinol can enhance appetite)
- Promethazine or ondansetron are frequently administered to treat nausea and vomiting.
- Neuropathy
- Pain
- Fluid retention

Total Parenteral Nutrition

Total parenteral feeding can be used in a variety of settings. Some of the most common include:

- Malnourishment due to any cause
- Liver or kidney failure
- Short bowel syndrome
- Severe burns

- Enterocutaneous fistulas

- Sepsis

- Chemotherapy and radiation

- Neonates

- Any disorder needing full bowel rest, such as pancreatitis, ulcerative colitis, or Crohn's disease.

Essentially, any situation in which the patient is unable to swallow or digest food via the stomach and intestines may necessitate the use of total parenteral nutrition. The goal is to keep the patient nourished while preventing wasting or malnutrition.

Possible Complications with Total Parenteral Nutrition

Although total parenteral nutrition is an efficient way to keep patients nourished when they are unable to eat on their own, various complications are likely, and physicians should regularly watch their patients to ensure that they do not develop one of the following conditions:

- Acidosis

- Calcification of the vena cava

- Electrolyte imbalances

- Glycemic imbalances, such as hyperglycemia or hypoglycemia

- Hematoma

- Liver dysfunction

- Pneumothorax

- Infection at the catheter site

- Triglyceride imbalances

Proper blood work monitoring will help to prevent or detect the majority of these illnesses, which can then be treated with medication or a different TPN formulation.

Sympathomimetic Agents

Sympathomimetic drugs mimic the body's natural sympathetic nervous response system, which produces transmitters such as adrenaline, norepinephrine, and dopamine. These medicines are widely used in emergency situations to treat cardiac arrest and shock. They are also used to treat extremely low blood pressure and prevent preterm labor. Many stimulants used to treat attention deficit disorder contain sympathomimetic characteristics.

Sympathomimetic drugs include of the following:

- Ephedrine

- Methylphenidate

- Pemoline

- Caffeine

- Dobutamine

- Dopamine
- Terbutaline

These medications may cause the following side effects:

- Hypertension
- Cardiac arrhythmia
- Nervousness
- Headache
- Anxiety
- Dilated pupils
- Vertigo

Benzodiazepines

Benzodiazepines stimulate the action of the neurotransmitter GABA, which causes a depressive effect on the central nervous system. While these medications eventually replaced the more lethal barbiturates, they remain associated with significant physical dependence and withdrawal symptoms. Benzodiazepines are used for sedation, hypnosis, and anticonvulsive treatment. Certain benzodiazepines are used to treat the symptoms of alcohol withdrawal. Most barbiturates are classified as Class IV prohibited substances. The most often used benzodiazepines are:

- Diazepam
- Lorazepam
- Clonazepam
- Alprazolam
- Midazolam
- Temazepam

Side effects of benzodiazepines include:

- Physical dependence
- Sedation
- Drowsiness
- Dizziness
- Lack of coordination

Methotrexate

Methotrexate is a drug used to treat severe psoriasis, rheumatoid arthritis, and certain types of cancer, including breast cancer, lung cancer, lymphoma, and leukemia.

Methotrexate belongs to a class of medicines known as antimetabolites. It works by reducing the growth of abnormal cells and disrupting immune system activity. Methotrexate has numerous side effects, some of which are potentially serious, including:

- Dizziness
- Drowsiness
- Headache
- Swollen gums
- Increased chance of infection
- Hair loss
- Confusion
- Weakness

Methotrexate is administered weekly and should not be taken on a daily basis. Dosing errors with methotrexate can be lethal. If you have a prescription for daily methotrexate, notify the pharmacist right away so that the doctor may be called. Signage at pharmacies reminding personnel of this dosing requirement can help to avoid dangerous errors.

Corticosteroids

Corticosteroids are a broad class of medications that treat a wide range of edema and inflammation-related conditions. Corticosteroids, while synthesized, are identical to naturally occurring cortisol. Corticosteroid medications can be taken orally as nasal sprays, eye and ear drops, topical lotions and ointments, inhalants, or injections. They are used to treat a variety of conditions, such as asthma, skin rashes, and arthritis.

Examples of commonly used corticosteroids are:

- Prednisone
- Hydrocortisone
- Triamcinolone
- Mometasone
- Budesonide
- Fluocinolone
- Betamethasone
- Dexamethasone

Corticosteroids can be dangerous if used for an extended period of time, especially when used topically. It may injure healthy tissues. Other adverse effects of corticosteroids include:

- Insulin resistance and diabetes
- Osteoporosis
- Depression
- Hypertension

- Hypothyroidism

Smoking Cessation

Smoking is a major cause of many serious ailments, including heart disease and cancer. Quitting smoking is one of the most important things you can do for your health; nonetheless, the challenges of overcoming a nicotine addiction are well known. In addition to ongoing support and behavioral treatment, medications like bupropion (Zyban) and varenicline (Chantix) can help people quit smoking. Additionally, nicotine replacement treatments such as gum, patches, and lozenges can help patients deal with cravings when quitting. When it comes to quitting smoking, friends and family provide the most powerful type of support.

Acetaminophen Dosage

The maximum daily dose of acetaminophen for adults with healthy livers is 4,000 mg. The maximum dose for people with impaired liver function due to alcoholism or liver disease is 2,000 mg per day or less. Some patients with hepatic dysfunction may be unable to take acetaminophen. Acetaminophen is primarily metabolized by the liver. When the liver is overwhelmed with acetaminophen, the pathways that metabolize it become saturated, the liver is unable to keep up, and the acetaminophen is digested via a different pathway. When this happens, the result is poisonous. The toxic substance accumulates in the liver, causing damage.

Alcohol and Medications

The majority of medications should be used without alcohol. Adverse effects vary depending on the medicine. Alcohol combined with medications can occasionally cause nausea and vomiting, fainting, loss of coordination, or extreme tiredness. A more severe reaction may result in cardiac problems, internal bleeding, and difficulty breathing. Some substances, when combined with alcohol, can create a dangerous combination. Alcohol is a potent CNS depressant. The combination of alcohol with other depressants, such as benzodiazepines or sleeping drugs, can be exceedingly harmful and cause patients to cease breathing. The combination of alcohol and acetaminophen can cause significant liver damage. When taking metronidazole, alcohol can cause serious side effects such as nausea, vomiting, and liver damage.

Hypertension and Medications

Many over-the-counter medications can cause an increase in blood pressure, which can be dangerous to patients with hypertension. Some of the pharmaceuticals known to be problematic for people with hypertension are NSAIDs such as ibuprofen and naproxen, decongestants such as pseudoephedrine, weight loss formulas and supplements, and caffeine-containing migraine medications. Patients with high blood pressure should see their physician or pharmacist before using any medications or herbal supplements. Symptoms of high blood pressure include headaches, dizziness, and shortness of breath. Instruct them to check their blood pressure on a regular basis. Take note of any significant changes and notify their doctor immediately.

Measurements and Calculations

Converting Teaspoon and Tablespoon Measurements into Milliliters

When delivering medications, a teaspoon equals 5 mL and a tablespoon is 15 mL.

The pharmacist should show patients how to properly give liquid medications with a specially approved spoon or oral syringe. Patients should be reminded not to administer medications with spoons made for food, despite the designations teaspoon and tablespoon, because sizes differ.

- 2 tsp. = 10 mL
- 2 tbsp. = 30 mL
- 4 tbsp. = 60 mL
- 1.5 tsp. = 7.5 mL
- 0.5 tbsp. = 7.5 mL
- 20 mL = 4 tsp.
- 2.5 mL = 0.5 tsp.

Converting Milliliters into Ounces

One liquid ounce is equal to 30 milliliters. Use a graduated cylinder to correctly measure liquid medications for dispensing. Pour gently.

- 180 mL = 6 ounces
- 240 mL = 8 ounces
- 90 mL = 3 ounces
- 2 ounces = 60 mL
- 12 ounces = 360 mL
- 5 ounces = 150 mL

Ratio of Cups to Pints to Quarts to Gallons

One pint equals two cups. There are two pints in a quart. One gallon equals four quarts. Because a cup contains eight ounces:

- One pint is 16 ounces.
- One quart is 32 ounces.
- One gallon is 128 ounces.

Conversion of Grams to Pounds

One kilogram (1000 grams) is equivalent to 2.2 pounds.

- 1 pound = 454 grams
- 2 pounds = 908 grams
- 227 grams = 0.5 pounds
- 681 grams = 1.5 pounds

Conversion of Grams to Ounces

A dry ounce is equivalent to 30 grams.

- 15 grams = 0.5 ounce
- 60 grams = 2 ounces
- 120 grams = 4 ounces
- 1.5 ounces = 45 grams
- 3 ounces = 90 grams

Conversion of Drops to Milliliters

Each mL contains 20 drops.

- 5 gtt ou bid x 10 days =10 ml (5 drops in each eye twice daily for 10 days)
- 1 gtt au tid x 30 days = 9 ml (1 drop in each ear three times daily for 30 days)
- 2 gtt os qd x 15 days = 1.5 mL (2 drops in left eye daily for 15 days)
- 1 gtt ou q2h x 5 days = 6 mL (1 drop in both eyes every 2 hours for 5 days)
- 3 gtt sl q4h x 7 days = 6.3 mL (3 drops sublingually every 4 hours for 7 days)

Most medications given as drops come in standard-sized bottles. The entire bottle is dispensed, even if it contains more than the required number of days' supply. It is still necessary to calculate days' supply for insurance purposes and to determine how many or which size bottle to use.

Conversion of Grains to Milligrams

One grain is equivalent to 65 milligrams.

- 2 grains = 130 mg
- 1.5 grains = 97.5 mg
- 0.5 grains = 32.5 mg
- 325 mg = 5 grains
- 650 mg = 10 grains
- 162.5 mg = 2.5 grains

Celsius and Fahrenheit Temperatures Conversions

The formula for converting Fahrenheit to Celsius is:

$$C = (F - 32) \times \frac{9}{5}$$

The formula for converting Celsius to Fahrenheit is:

$$F = C \times \left(\frac{9}{5}\right) + 32$$

Examples:

40°F	=	4.45°C
67°F	=	19.46°C
98.6°F	=	37°C
102°F	=	38.89°C
10°C	=	50°F
50°C	=	122F

Pediatric Dose Rules

Young's rule relies on age to calculate the dose, using the formula

$$\text{adult dose} \times \left(\frac{\text{age}}{\text{age}+12}\right) = \text{pediatric dose}$$

Drilling's rule also relies on age. The formula used in this rule is

$$\frac{\text{age} \times \text{adult dose}}{12} = \text{pediatric dose}$$

Fried's rule uses the child's age in months, with the formula

$$\frac{\text{age in months} \times \text{adult dose}}{150} = \text{pediatric dose}$$

Clark's rule is based on the child's weight in pounds, using the formula

$$\frac{\text{weight in pounds} \times \text{adult dose}}{150} = \text{pediatric dose}$$

Proportional Calculation

Proportional calculations are extensively used in pharmacies. They are used for determining how much medication to dispense, calculating a dose, and compounding. A proportional computation is typically constructed as:

$$\frac{a}{b} = \frac{c}{d}$$

In a basic situation, the technician could have been given the following prescription: Amoxicillin suspension, 250 mg every 10 hours. When I examined the shelf, the only accessible concentration was 200 mg/5 mL. Create an equation to compute the dose.

$$\frac{200\,mg}{5\,ml} = \frac{250\,mg}{x}$$

To find x, multiply 5 by 250 and divide by 200. The answer is 6.25 milliliters. When performing these calculations, ensure that you use the same units of measurement. If one side is in mg/ml and the other is in mcg/ml, the calculations will be incorrect. To verify that the units are the same, one must be altered.

Proportion Technique

To solve dilution problems with the proportion technique, follow these steps:

- Setting up your proportion equation:

$$\left(\frac{x}{total}\right) = \left(\frac{percentage}{100}\right)$$

- Solve for x for the total number of units of active ingredient in the solution.
- Determine the quantity of diluted solution to be made using proportions:

$$\frac{active\ ingredient}{x} = \frac{desired\ dilution\ percentage}{100}$$

- Solve for x to get the total quantity of diluted solution you can make.
- Determine how much diluent to add by subtracting the original amount of solution you had from the total amount of diluted solution.

Explain how to use the proportion technique to calculate dilutions of solutions and solve the following problem: How much sterile water would be required to dilute one liter of 70% alcohol solution to 40% solution? How much of a 40% solution would you create?

To solve the problem:

$$\frac{x\,ml}{1000\,ml} = \frac{70}{100}$$

Solve for x:

$$\frac{1000 \times 70}{100} = x$$

The solution contains 700 ml of alcohol.

$$\frac{700}{x} = \frac{40}{100}$$

Solve for x:

$$\frac{700 \times 100}{40} = x$$

The total amount of diluted solution that can be made is 1750 ml. To get this solution, add 750 ml of sterile water.

V/V, W/W, and W/V Concentrations

Concentrations can be stated as a ratio of substances or a percentage. In concentrations, V/V, W/W, and W/V are used to express solute (drug) to solvent ratios.

V/V denotes a volume/volume ratio, and the unit of measurement is mL.

W/W is a weight/weight ratio, and the unit of measurement is grams.

W/V stands for weight/volume ratio, and the unit of measurement is grams per milliliter.

1. V/V = 1:200 = 1 ml/200 ml = 0.5%

2. W/W = 3:100 = 3 grams/100 grams = 3%

3. W/V = 15/100 = 15 grams/100 ml = 15%

Alligation Method

The alligation strategy is sometimes known as the "Tic-Tac-Toe" method because the problems are placed on a grid resembling a tic-tac-toe board. Set up the problem by putting the desired concentration in the middle box, the highest concentration in the upper left corner, and the lowest concentration in the bottom left. Move from the lower left to the upper right corner. The difference between the numbers in the lower left and middle boxes is displayed in the top right corner. Moving from the upper left to the lower right corner, the difference between the numbers in the upper left and middle is displayed in the lower right corner. The number on the right represents the percentage of the concentration across from it on the left used to produce the desired concentration. Proportion math will help you determine how much of each to use.

Problem

The pharmacist has instructed you to mix 0.75 L of a 70% alcohol solution with 1.5L of a 40% alcohol solution. Show the strength of the final solution. This type of problem is referred to as a $C_1 V_1 = C_2 V_2$ problem, with C standing for concentration and V standing for volume.

The numbers refer to each solution in the combination. Set up the equation to solve the problem as:

$$C_1V_1 + C_2V_2 = C_FV_F$$

To solve the problem, set up the equation as follows:

$$0.7 \, (750 \text{ ml}) + 0.4 \, (1500 \text{ ml}) = C_F(2250 \text{ ml})$$

Solve the problem for C_F:

$$525 \text{ ml} + 600 \text{ ml} = C_F(2250 \text{ ml})$$

$$\frac{1125}{2250} = C_F$$

$$C_F = 0.5$$

Which means the strength of the finished solution will be 50%.

Sample Algebra Problems

1 Sample

If a patient comes in with a prescription for 30 tablets of 50 mg Zoloft at a wholesale price of $4 a tablet, how much would the script cost after a 50% markup and a $3 dispensing fee?

Solution

First determine the total wholesale price:

$4 x 30 = $120.

Now, add in the markup,

$120 x 1.50 = $180

Add in your dispensing fee,

$180 + $3 = $183

$183 is the total retail price for 30 tablets of 50 mg Zoloft.

If you work in a pharmacy and sell 30 10 mg Norvasc tablets for $110, and you know your average markup is 40% above wholesale, plus a $6 dispensing fee per prescription, what is the wholesale price your pharmacy pays for each Norvasc tablet?

Solution

To solve this problem, begin by subtracting the dispensing fee from the total:

$110 – $6 = $104.

To reverse the markup, divide $104 by 1.40 (the 1 in 1.40 represents the 100% of the markup price)

$104 ÷ 1.40 = $74.28.

Now divide by the quantity, $74.28 by 30

$74.28 ÷ 30 = $2.47.

Your pharmacy is paying $2.47 for each tablet of 10 mg Norvasc.

Durable vs. Non-Durable Medical Equipment

Durable medical equipment is any non-disposable gadget used to treat a medical condition. Wheelchairs, walkers, diabetic blood testing monitors, home oxygen devices, nebulizers, prostheses, slings, braces, and orthotics are all examples of medical equipment.

Non-durable medical equipment is defined as a product designed to treat a medical problem but intended to be discarded or used just once. Diabetes supplies include lancets, test strips, insulin syringes, needles, casts, catheters, and ostomy equipment.

Blood Pressure Monitors

The general public has access to several blood pressure monitors. Standard cuffs for the arm and wrist are offered. Some cuffs automatically inflate, while others need to be manually inflated. Advanced blood pressure monitors not only inflate automatically, but also save your readings so you and your doctor can easily view and track them. Most experts believe that upper arm monitors are more accurate than wrist monitors. Readings on wrist monitors can vary greatly depending on the position of the arm and wrist, so read and follow the manufacturer's recommendations for use. A patient can test the accuracy of a wrist monitor by bringing it to a doctor's appointment and measuring his or her blood pressure using both the wrist monitor and the doctor's equipment.

Orthopedic Supplies

Braces, crutches, splints, insoles, and other things fall under the category of orthopedic goods. Most of these devices are intended to position and stabilize the injured body part in order to facilitate healing or avoid harm. Knee and ankle braces are two typical choices for this purpose. Wrist and thumb braces can help treat and prevent illnesses such as carpal tunnel syndrome. A sling or splint may be required to limit mobility and promote healing after a shattered limb. Crutches help patients with leg, ankle, or foot injuries keep weight off the damaged area.

Ostomy Supplies

Ostomy supplies are used following surgery to relocate a part of the colon or bladder. The ostomy supplies include adhesive wafers, skin protectants, deodorants, and waste collection bags. Patients with ostomies will have a stoma in their body. To collect waste products, a collecting bag with an adhesive ring (also known as a wafer) is applied to the skin around the stoma. Many of these products are accessible at pharmacies or can be ordered specifically for patients. It is vital to determine which type of ostomy surgery a patient has had (colostomy, urostomy, or ileostomy) so that the necessary supplies may be ordered.

Insulin Pump

Some people with Type 1 diabetes struggle to control their blood sugar levels and may need frequent insulin injections. For these people, an insulin pump that provides constant insulin infusion throughout the day is preferred to several injections, which can cause blood sugar highs and lows. An insulin pump is made up of numerous parts and supplies, including the pump itself, an insulin reservoir, a subcutaneous cannula, and a tube system. The reservoir, cannula, and tubing system are replaceable and may be purchased at many pharmacies or online. The doctor programs insulin pumps to provide precise doses of insulin at certain intervals in order to keep the patient's blood sugar levels stable.

Crash Cart

A crash cart, also known as a code cart, is a cart that is positioned in various sections of hospitals or other medical facilities to be used in the event of a cardiac or other emergency requiring resuscitation. The crash cart contains medical supplies and medications necessary for resuscitation, including:

- Heart rate monitors
- Defibrillators
- Medications used during intubation include succinylcholine (paralytic), etomidate, midazolam, or other sedatives.
- Advanced Cardiac Life Support. Medications including amiodarone, atropine, dopamine, epinephrine, lidocaine, sodium bicarbonate, and vasopressin
- Other medications that may be added include adenosine, dextrose, diazepam, naloxone, and nitroglycerin.

Code Blue

Code Blue is used in many hospitals and medical facilities across the country to indicate a medical emergency requiring immediate resuscitation. The most common reason for a Code Blue call is cardiac or respiratory arrest. Code Blue, along with the patient's exact location, is broadcast across the hospital intercom system. This is an indication that emergency personnel should come on the location as soon as possible. A pharmacist and a technician are normally assigned to respond to a Code Blue. Responsibilities will vary depending on location, therefore educate yourself with the policies in place. If supplies run short, pharmacy professionals may need to bring additional medication or call for more. Following a Code Blue, technicians will be dispatched to refill the crash cart.

Intubation

Intubation involves putting a tube into the trachea via the mouth or nose. In an emergency, it may be accomplished with a tracheotomy or other surgical procedures. Intubation is used for a variety of purposes.

- To maintain an open airway
- To administer some types of medication
- To facilitate lung ventilation

- To prevent asphyxiation

Intubation is an intrusive and uncomfortable procedure, thus certain medications are supplied during it. Succinylcholine is used as a paralytic, as are sedatives such as midazolam and etomidate. Intubation is often performed under general anesthesia, however it can be done while the patient is awake if necessary.

CPR

Cardiopulmonary resuscitation (CPR) is an emergency procedure that assists patients who are not breathing or whose hearts have stopped beating. The compressions mimic heartbeats, which help to keep blood moving throughout the body and prevent brain damage until the heart can restart. Artificial respiration pushes air into the lungs. The goal of CPR is not to restart the heart, but rather to keep the tissue from dying and maximize the person's chances of survival. Adults use a compression ratio of 30 to 2 breaths. The ratio in children is 15:2. The abbreviation CAB could help you recall the order of compressions, airway, and breathing. Perform 100 compressions per minute at a depth of about 5 cm. All healthcare workers should get and maintain CPR certification on a biannual basis.

Heimlich Maneuver

The Heimlich Maneuver is performed to assist people who are choking. The movement helps remove food or other things that have been trapped in the airway. The technique is as follows:

- Stand behind the victim, wrapping your arms around them.
- Making a fist, position the thumb side of the fist so that it is pressing into the abdomen, above the navel and below the rib cage.
- With the other hand, quickly thrust the fist upward, slamming it into the upper abdomen.
- Repeat until the object is expelled.
- Heimlich Maneuver training is frequently included in CPR classes.

Standard Hospital Emergency Codes

While there is no standard structure for hospitals, several issues may develop in hospitals and medical institutions. It is vital to understand the codes used to identify certain situations and your role in them, if they emerge.

Some choices are:

- **Code Blue** – often used to identify a cardiac or respiratory emergency
- **Bomb threat** – keep the caller on the phone while contacting security
- **Child abduction** – often identified by Amber Alert or Code Pink. Staff may be assigned to monitor a specific exit.
- **Combative person** – a team may be assembled to present a show of force
- **Fire** – often identified as Code Red. Know the nearest exit and route.

Pharmacy Laws and Regulations

HIPAA

The Health Insurance Portability and Accountability Act (HIPAA), passed in 1996, went into effect in 2003. The act's goal is to protect patients' medical information from improper distribution while still allowing for distribution in specific circumstances. HIPAA requires healthcare personnel to do the following:

- Employ a designated privacy officer
- Create a method to effectively secure protected information.
- Establish HIPAA-compliant privacy policies
- Advise patients of their rights under HIPAA and how to request their own health information
- Advise patients on how to make a complaint if their privacy is infringed.
- Train employees how to properly maintain patient privacy
- Employees who fail to comply with HIPAA standards and procedures may face sanctions.

Preparing Medications

Confidentiality is a top priority in patient care. As you prepare drugs, you may consult with the pharmacist or offer extra patient information. Although the drugstore layout may not provide for a good view of the waiting area, patients will most likely hear what you say. Discussing patient and prescription information in a setting where others may hear is not only a breach of trust and potentially embarrassing for the patient, but it is also a serious violation of HIPAA.

Patient Identifiable Information

Patient identifying information includes any information that can be used to identify a patient. This can include:

- Name
- Patient ID number
- Address
- Phone number
- Social security number

All interactions involving patient identifying information should take place in the most private setting possible. Paperwork containing this information must be kept out of the sight of other patients or anybody who does not have a legitimate reason to see it. Computers containing this information must be password protected and configured so that they are not visible to other patients or the general public.

Releasing Confidential Patient Information

Confidential patient information may be released in the following conditions:

- To other professionals involved in the patient's treatment, so that care can be efficiently coordinated.
- To third parties, medical and otherwise, when accompanied by a patient-signed release of information.
- To a third party payer in order to receive correct payment
- When requested by the patient for his or her personal use via a signed release of information.
- To public health professionals where the information constitutes a concern to public health, such as in cases of certain contagious diseases or dog attacks.
- By subpoena in certain circumstances

The Joint Commission

The Joint Commission is a non-profit, independent organization that certifies and accredits healthcare organizations throughout the United States, including hospitals. The Joint Commission (TJC) was formerly known as the Joint Commission for Accreditation of Healthcare Organizations (JCAHO).The Joint Commission accreditation is generally recognized throughout the United States as the highest standard for quality care. The Joint Commission's aim is to ensure that all patients receive the highest quality care at all hospitals across the country. This is accomplished by regular inspections of healthcare facilities, including pharmacies.

Facilities that fail to meet The Joint Commission's requirements must either comply with the suggestions given within a set deadline or be examined.

Food and Drug Administration (FDA)

The FDA is the Food and Drug Administration, and it was founded in 1927 to oversee the production and safety of food and drugs in the United States. The FDA's aim is to protect and promote public health by overseeing and regulating the manufacturing of the following:

- Food products
- Prescription medications
- Over-the-counter medications
- Tobacco products
- Dietary supplements
- Vaccines
- Biological drug products
- Blood transfusions
- Medical devices

- Cosmetics

The FDA's director is the Commissioner of Food and Drugs, who is appointed by the President. The FDA's Office of Criminal Investigations investigates and enforces food and medicine safety regulations. The Food, Drug, and Cosmetic Act contains the vast majority of the legislation that governs and influences FDA activities.

Federal Food, Drug, and Cosmetic Act

The Food and Drug Administration (FDA) was founded under the Federal Food, Drug, and Cosmetic Act (FD&C) to ensure the safety of food, pharmaceuticals, and cosmetics. The FD&C Act was passed in 1938 in response to an incident in which over 100 individuals died after taking a medication that included residues of diethylene glycol. The Act has been updated multiple times throughout the years to suit changing technology.

Drug Enforcement Administration (DEA)

The Drug Enforcement Administration (DEA) is a government entity founded in 1973.Its goal, according to the Controlled Substances Act, is to police drug laws and combat drug smuggling. The DEA frequently shares authority with Immigration and Customs Enforcement and the Federal Bureau of Investigation. The DEA's principal goals are to:

- Educate the public through youth and community-based programs to help reduce demand for illicit and diverted narcotics.

- Encourage state and local law enforcement efforts to decrease drug-related crime and violence.

- Break up sources and suppliers of illegal and diverted drugs, both local and foreign

Prescription Drug Marketing Act

The Prescription Drug Marketing Act was signed into law in 1988.The Act has two objectives:

- To ensure that all pharmaceuticals offered to consumers are both safe and effective.

- To protect consumers from counterfeit, misbranded, adulterated, expired, or subpotent medications.

The Prescription Drug Amendments, passed in 1992, amended the Act. Before the Prescription Drug Marketing Act, there were numerous reports of pharmaceutical safety and efficacy difficulties. Medication diversion was a major problem, with medications sold that were not meant for transfer, such as pharmaceutical samples and previously exported drugs.

USP-NF

The US Pharmacopeia and National Formulary are published together in a format known as the USP/NF. All medications distributed in the United States, whether prescription or over-the-counter, must meet the USP-NF standards. The USP regulates and establishes standards for medications, foods, and dietary supplements. The USP creates pharmaceutical information, including drug use details, and distributes it to healthcare decision-makers including practitioners and pharmacists. One example is the mechanism used by Medicare Prescription

Drug Benefit Plans to create formularies. Many other countries have chosen to adopt the United States' USP rather than developing their own.

U.S. NRC

The United States Nuclear Regulatory Committee was created in 1975.The primary purpose of the United States Nuclear Regulatory Commission is to create laws that assure radiation safety. The NRC is in charge of creating standards for nuclear reactor safety, radioactive waste disposal, and nuclear medicine. The NRC ensures that patients receive the proper and acceptable radiation dose to treat their sickness, and that radioactive substances used in nuclear medicine are appropriately controlled, stored, and disposed of after use. The NRC also oversees the training of pharmacists and personnel who work with nuclear medications.

CDC

The term "CDC" refers to the Centers for Disease Control and Prevention. The Centers for Disease Control and Prevention (CDC) is a government entity founded during World War II to help prevent and control the spread of dangerous diseases. The CDC's aim is to educate and enlighten the public so that they can make more informed health-care decisions. They work with local health agencies to get information to as many people as possible. In addition to communicable diseases, the CDC looks into chronic illnesses, disabilities, occupational and environmental health concerns, obesity, birth defects, and bioterrorism.

Compounding and Manufacturing Medications

The FDA distinguishes between compounding and manufacturing. Compounding includes creating patient-specific medicine doses as prescribed by a physician, whereas manufacturing involves mass-producing non-patient-specific drugs. Federal legislation allows for compounding, but not manufacturing, on pharmacy premises. Pharmacies violate the statute allowing compounding when:

- Compound drugs ahead of time in anticipation of prescriptions
- Compound drugs from ingredients that have been withdrawn from market
- Compound drugs from ingredients not approved by the FDA
- Compound drugs using commercial scale manufacturing or testing equipment
- Compound drugs for third-party resale
- Compound drug that are otherwise commercially available

FDA Process of Drug Approval

Drug approval is a difficult process that takes an average of twelve years. Companies assess their medications internally for around four years before submitting them to the FDA for human trials. After the FDA permits testing, the drug undergoes three steps of human testing:

- **Phase one** lasts approximately a year and involves 80 to 100 healthy volunteers. The drug's safety is being studied at this time.
- **Phase two** lasts about two years and involves 100 to 300 patient participants. The purpose of phase two is to test the drug's efficacy.

- **Phase three** takes approximately three years. During this time, around 1000 to 3000 individuals in hospitals and clinics will get the medication as part of the testing procedure, while efficacy and side effects are thoroughly investigated.

After the testing is finished, an application is submitted to the FDA for review. After the FDA has authorized the new medicine, doctors can prescribe it.

Recording of Distributed Prescription Medications and Controlled Substances

Pharmacies are required to keep a log or other record of prescriptions dispensed. The prescription must be on file for at least five years. The record or file must always be available for review by the pharmacy board and other authorities. Records of administered medications must include the following information:

- Date dispensed
- Drug name, strength, and dosage form
- Patient's name
- Quantity dispensed
- Patient's address

When filing prescriptions that have been filled, **CII medications** should have their own file, **CIII – CV prescriptions** should have their own file, and other prescription medications should have their own file.

DEA Controlled Substances

- **CI** – These substances have no recognized medicinal utility, have a high potential for abuse, and have not been shown safe even when provided under medical supervision. Examples include heroin and LSD.
- **CII** – These compounds have been approved for medical applications (though there may be considerable limitations) and have a high misuse potential. Abuse may cause physical or psychological dependence. Examples include oxycodone and methadone.
- **CIII** – Although there is a risk of abuse, it is lower than that of CI and CII medicines. These compounds have medicinal applications. Physical or psychological reliance is possible. Examples include ketamine and codeine.
- **CIV** – Abuse potential exists, but it is lower than that of CIII substances. These substances have accepted medical uses. Limited physical or psychological dependence is possible. Examples include diazepam and zolpidem.
- **CV** – These medicines have a low abuse risk. These medications have legitimate medical applications. It is possible to have a limited physical or psychological dependency. Cough suppressants include pregabalin and low-dose codeine.

Valid Controlled Substances Prescription

A genuine and lawful prescription for restricted pharmaceuticals must contain all of the following:

- Patient's full name and address

- Date written
- Prescriber's name, address, and DEA number
- Drug name, dosage form, and strength
- Prescribed quantity
- Directions for use
- Refills authorized, if any
- Handwritten signature of the prescriber (or e-signature if transmitted electronically)

If a prescription comes at the pharmacy without any of this information, the pharmacist must contact the prescriber to clarify the details. A physician may provide verbal authorization over the phone for a missing signature unless the prescription is for a prohibited substance. In this case, the prescription must be returned for a physical signature.

CII Medication Faxed or Ordered Verbally

For a CII prescription to be faxable, the patient must be one of the following:
- A resident in a long-term care facility
- A resident in community-based care
- Enrolled as a patient in a hospice program
- The recipient of compounded home infusion or IV pain therapy

The fax must include the prescriber's signature. The fax will serve as the written prescription document.

Verbal instructions for CII drugs are only accepted in an emergency. The amount of medication administered is limited to what is necessary during an emergency. The clinician must write a prescription for the emergency quantity and mail or deliver it to the pharmacy within seven days.

Maintaining Inventory of CII Medications

CII medications must be stored in a separate room from other prescriptions, particularly CIII-CV pharmaceuticals. A perpetual inventory of CII medications must be kept, with each pill carefully documented in a ledger. Every quarter, the perpetual inventory must be reconciled to the pharmacy's computerized inventory system. Furthermore, prescriptions for CII medications must be filled separately from other prescriptions. It is never authorized to store CII medications outside of the sealed security cabinet. Many hospitals have a dedicated opioid division where all orders are prepared.

Changes to a CII Prescription

Before modifying a CII prescription, the pharmacist must tell the prescriber. Only a pharmacist may accept the prescriber's changes.
- Dosage form, for example capsule vs. tablet
- Strength of the medication
- Quantity of the medication

- Directions

Even after a phone call to the doctor, the following alterations are not permitted:

- Changes to the patient's name
- Change to a different controlled substance
- Addition of the prescriber's signature, if it was forgotten

If these changes are required, the patient must return the prescription to the prescriber to obtain a new and exact prescription.

CII Medications Transferred

To order CII medications from a wholesale warehouse, the pharmacy must appropriately fill out the DEA Form 222, either on paper or electronically. Electronic forms must be stored in a way that enables for inspection if needed. The DEA Form 222 must specify the date, drugs "ordered," and quantity. The pharmacy must also use the DEA Form 222 when transferring or returning CII medications to the wholesaler.

It is imperative to adhere to the following regulations concerning DEA Form 222:

- The form is not editable. If an error occurs, the person filling out the form must start over.
- The green copy of the DEA Form 222 is sent to the local DEA office.
- The blue copy of the form must be maintained on file at the pharmacy for a minimum of two years.

Prescriptions Expiration and Refills

Refills are not permitted for medications designated as CII. They are considered to be timeless. The pharmacist has the responsibility to exercise professional discretion in determining whether or not to dispense the prescribed medication. Medications categorized as CIII-CV are limited to a maximum of five refills. The prescription remains valid for a duration of six months starting from the date of issuance, or until it has been refilled five times, whichever occurs earlier. Unscheduled drugs may qualify for unlimited (or as needed) refills. The prescription will become invalid after one year from the date it was written.

DEA Numbers

DEA numbers adhere to a highly precise formula. To ascertain the authenticity of a DEA number, verify if it conforms to this specific pattern:

- DEA numbers start with two letters, followed by six numbers and a "check" digit.
- The first letter of the DEA number represents the type of practitioner. For example, B denotes a hospital or clinic provider, C a practitioner, and E a manufacturer.
- Add the first, third and fifth digit. This is sum A.
- Add the second, fourth and sixth digit, and multiply that answer by two. This is sum B.
- Add Sum A and Sum B.
- The last digit in your answer should match the check digit at the end of the DEA number.

Restricted Drug Distribution Programs

1. **Thalidomide** uses the program **S.T.E.P.S.** (System for Thalidomide Education and Prescribing Safety). Patients must register, undergo pregnancy testing (if applicable), and receive mandatory counseling before receiving their first medicine. Before obtaining any further drugs, eligible patients must undergo regular pregnancy testing and mandatory counseling.

2. **Isotretinoin** employs the iPledge program to limit drug distribution. Before receiving their first prescription, patients must register with the program, undergo pregnancy testing (if applicable), agree to use two methods of birth control, and attend all scheduled appointments. Female patients must first complete monthly pregnancy tests before logging into the iPledge system to detail their birth control methods and respond to program-related questions.

3. **Clozapine** prescriptions necessitate the use of a program to monitor the patient's white blood cell count as well as his or her absolute neutrophil level. Different manufacturers have their own plans, and any of them are appropriate as long as the doctor and pharmacist can monitor the patient's response to the medication.

Drug Diversion

Drug diversion is a serious concern in the healthcare system. Drug diversion is described as the use of medication for purposes other than those intended. This can happen at several levels:

- Health care practitioners may divert medications from stock for personal use.

- Patients may seek medications and then sell them to others.

- People may steal medications from the person to whom it was prescribed.

Each of them is a case of drug diversion. Many measures are in place at the pharmacy level to prevent drug diversion, such as requiring identification, double counting regulated drugs, and maintaining a continuous CII inventory log. Opiates (oxycodone and hydrocodone), stimulants (methylphenidate), and depressants (diazepam and lorazepam) are the most commonly diverted medications. Pseudoephedrine is a commonly diverted medication in many places because it is used to produce methamphetamine.

Forged Prescription

When drug users falsify or modify prescriptions, they often do so incorrectly, making it simpler to identify. When receiving prescriptions, always look for these common "tells":

- The drug seeker may provide personal information that is contradictory.

- The prescription could be prepared on a form by a doctor who does not frequently prescribe this type of medication, such as cardiologists or other specialists. This could indicate stolen prescription blanks.

- Errors with "sig" abbreviations are frequently a "tell," such as a drug that obviously does not match the customary dose (e.g., OxyContin q4h instead of bid) or simple errors with the codes (1 qbid).

- Errors in dosing may appear.

- Clear erasures of quantities or refills can be a giveaway. Always confirm a prescription that appears to have been changed by deleting.
- Two different types of ink may indicate changes made to an otherwise valid prescription.
- Refills on CII drugs can be a red flag, but they can also be caused by a faulty prescription. Confirm with the prescriber.
- Watch quantity numbers carefully.

Mailing a Prescription

Certain pharmacies provide the service of delivering drugs to patients. The kind of prescriptions that can be sent by mail differ from state to state, so it is important to verify the regulations in your area before delivering any medications. Prescriptions should be sent via mail using a dedicated padded envelope. By inserting cotton into the pill bottle, the pills can be safeguarded and the likelihood of their being damaged can be minimized. If you work in a brick-and-mortar pharmacy and the pills are being sent by mail as a gesture of goodwill to the customer, please instruct them to prevent any instances of missed medications or misunderstandings.

FDA Recall Classes I, II, and III

The FDA employs a tripartite classification system to ascertain the severity of drug recalls.
- **Class I** recalls are the most serious. Drugs affected by a class I recall are likely to cause serious adverse health conditions or death.
- **Class II** recalls are slightly less serious. While the possibilities of death or serious health consequences are unlikely, temporary health problems may occur because of taking the drug.
- **Class III** recalls are used when a drug has violated an FDA regulation, but adverse health consequences are unlikely to occur.

Additional recall measures that may take place involve FDA Market Withdrawals, when a minor violation arises and either the problem is resolved or the product is removed from the market.

Medical equipment is susceptible to recalls referred to as FDA Medical Device Safety Alerts.

Disposing of Medications

The FDA has provided the following guidelines for the disposal of pharmaceuticals:
- Do not dump drugs down the toilet unless the box clearly states so.
- If there are community take-back initiatives in your region, take advantage of them.
- Before putting drugs in the trash, they should:
- Be removed from their original containers and mixed with a substance such as old coffee grounds or cat litter,
- Be placed in a sealed bag or other empty container to prevent leakage.
- Before disposing of a medication container, destroy the label or make it unreadable.

Ask a pharmacist for more information on proper drug disposal.

General Duties of a Certified Pharmacy Technician

Certified pharmacy technologists bear the majority of responsibilities in a retail drugstore. Some of the duties comprise:

- Accepting prescription orders from patients
- Checking the fax or computerized system for medication orders.
- Processing orders using pharmacy software
- Selecting correct products and counting or pouring medications to prepare the order
- Printing and attaching prescription labels
- Maintaining patient profiles
- File insurance claims and follow up on continuing insurance issues.
- Completing transactions at the cash register
- Answering phones
- Maintaining stock and inventory in the pharmacy

Pharmacy technicians are not authorized to provide medical advice to patients. Pharmacy technicians should remain informed about current drug and healthcare knowledge. Additionally, they should actively identify and report any potential errors or issues to the pharmacist.

Pharmacy Work Environments

Pharmacy technicians are employed in many pharmacy environments. Several establishments that employ skilled pharmacy technicians include:

- Retail pharmacy stores
- Hospitals
- Long-term care facilities
- Mail order pharmacies
- Medical supply stores

The working hours of pharmacy technologists may vary based on the employer. Although certain technicians adhere to a 9-to-5 schedule from Monday to Friday, numerous retail and hospital pharmacies operate continuously. Pharmacy technicians are frequently required to be available on weekends and holidays as necessary. A significant number of pharmacy technologists are members of professional unions.

Ratio of Pharmacy Technicians to Pharmacists

The regulations vary regarding the specific ratio of technicians to pharmacists permitted at any given time. Certain states establish a suggested ratio, while others enforce it as a legal requirement. Certain states require a 2:1 ratio, while others permit a 3:1 ratio. By maintaining a modest ratio of technicians to pharmacists, it becomes possible for pharmacists to properly manage technicians. Insufficient availability of pharmacists relative to an excess of technicians poses challenges in ensuring rigorous verification of prescriptions and prepared drugs prior to dispensing.

General Duties of a Certified Pharmacy Technician in a Hospital

In a hospital setting, pharmacy technicians are likely to accomplish the following:

- Goods maintenance includes ordering goods, storing inventory, removing expired inventory, and processing returns.
- Tracking and maintaining narcotic inventory
- Assist the pharmacist in preparing intravenous (IV) solutions and other sterile combinations, such as chemotherapeutic drugs and parenteral nutrition.
- Selecting the correct medication to fill orders
- Preparing medication for dispensing throughout the hospital
- Checking other technicians' work, depending on local laws
- Medication is delivered to hospital units and nursing floors on a planned and as-needed basis.
- Maintain drug delivery systems, such as automated dispensing equipment.
- Updating and maintaining patient profiles
- Maintaining the cleanliness of the pharmacy
- Assisting with the training of new technicians

Dispensing of Medication

In most hospitals, the nursing station acts as the focal point for each sector. It is where nurses go to get information and orders for the day. Automatic dispensing systems are typically encountered in nursing stations. If the hospital employs a pneumatic tube system, each nurses' station will most likely include a tube stop. The pharmacy technician fills the dispensing device or administers individual doses through the tubes. Nurses remove and deliver medications in accordance with medical instructions. It is vital that nurses adhere to the same pharmaceutical storage requirements as the pharmacy. Occasionally, training is conducted to ensure that rules are followed consistently throughout the facility. Pharmacy technicians may be dispatched to inspect the space to ensure that drugs are stored in conformity with applicable laws and hospital standards.

Dress Codes for Technicians

Many pharmacies enforce tight dress requirements for pharmacy technicians. Retail pharmacies often require business casual clothes to present a professional image, whereas hospital pharmacies prioritize safety and cleanliness. Depending on the area of the pharmacy where the technician works, one of the following may be necessary:

- Scrubs
- Foot covers
- Hair bonnets
- Masks
- Goggles or other eye coverings

Shoes in the drugstore must be closed toed. This is not only for hygiene reasons, but it is also an important safety precaution, especially when working with needles and syringes that can slip out of your grasp.

Cleaning Items Used to Count Medication

As work in the pharmacy advances, the tools used to measure, count, and pour medication may become dusty or contaminated with pharmaceutical dust. Counting trays, spatulas, and other measuring tools should be cleaned with hot soapy water at least once a day. Keep cleaning wipes on hand throughout the day so you may wipe down counting trays when necessary. After counting allergy-prone medications such as penicillin or sulfa antibiotics, clean the trays and spatulas well. Powder from these prescriptions may contaminate other medications tallied on the same equipment, resulting in an allergic reaction. To facilitate this, some pharmacies have separate counting trays for different prescriptions. After pouring or scooping liquid or cream medications, promptly clean the utensils used.

Areas of the Pharmacy to Be Cleaned Every Day

A pharmacy technician is responsible for keeping the drugstore clean. The drugstore should be clean as feasible. Dusting should happen on a regular basis. The daily cleaning tasks include:

- Wiping down the counter and all surface areas
- Clean all tools needed to deliver drugs.
- Cleaning keyboards and all phone surfaces
- Removing rubbish from the pharmacy.
- Sweeping or vacuuming the floor of the pharmacy
- Wet-mopping the pharmacy floor with disinfectant.
- Clean the lobby or waiting area seating with disinfectant, and sweep and wet-mop or vacuum the space.

Preceptor

Pharmacy preceptors teach and mentor pharmacy trainees. To hire interns or trainees, pharmacists must first become preceptor certified. While preceptor requirements vary depending on local legislation, the following are typically required:

- One to two years of full-time employment as a pharmacist in the location where they intend to be a preceptor.

- Fully licensed and maintaining good standing with the local Board of Pharmacy

- Willingness and desire to mentor students

- Willingness and motivation to conduct honest appraisals of students' ability.

- Willingness to allow students to evaluate their job as a preceptor.

State Board of Pharmacy

Each state has its own board of pharmacy. The board of pharmacy, a division of the state health department, licenses pharmacies, pharmacists, and technicians. Other exact functions may differ by state. The ultimate goal is to improve public health and safety by ensuring that all pharmacies in the state follow the same set of high standards. The board of pharmacy also acts as a liaison between the general public, pharmacies, and state government agencies. The state board of pharmacy inspects and evaluates pharmacies to verify that they meet the necessary requirements.

NABP

The NABP stands for the National Association of Pharmacy Boards. The organization's aim is to assist and support the various state boards of pharmacy. They are intended to ensure impartiality and help keep standards as consistent as possible among states. The NABP also supports the transfer of pharmacist licenses between states. The organization was founded in 1904.The NABP promotes pharmacy standards and evaluates pharmacist competency through examinations. The NABP's primary goal is to promote and protect public safety.

SDS

SDS (formerly MSDS) stands for Safety Data Sheets. These sections (available online with a subscription) provide information on a variety of materials and chemical substances, including physical attributes and spill procedures. Every pharmacy should have an SDS book (or internet access) immediately available in case of an accident. This is an OSHA requirement. The SDS provides the following specific information:

- Manufacturer

- Contractor information

- Identified dangers depending on routes of entrance.

- Potential for carcinogenicity or other hazards

- Potential for a fire or explosion, and ways for extinguishing if flammable.

- First aid treatment

- Clean up requirements

- Recommended safety equipment

- Directions for disposal

Chemical Spill

In the event of a chemical leak, adhere to the comprehensive spill response plan provided in the pharmacy. In general, the approach will include the following steps:

- Everyone in the spill area should be immediately warned and, if necessary, evacuated.
- Discard contaminated clothing and rinse any skin that has come into contact with the chemical.
- To learn more about the spilled chemical's flammability and volatility, consult the Safety Data Sheet.
- Don personal protective equipment, including respiratory protection, if needed.
- Use the absorption spill kit to clean up small or medium spills. You should know where this kit is at your pharmacy.
- For large spills, outside help may be required. Follow local procedures and policies.
- Once the spill has been absorbed, dispose of it in appropriate chemical spill bags.
- Decontaminate the area with water and detergent when appropriate.
- Report spills to supervisor.

Hazardous Waste

Pharmacies can generate considerable amounts of hazardous waste. The following materials are considered hazardous waste in pharmacies:
- Expired medications
- Medicines that were wrongly compounded
- Chemotherapy
- Products contaminated with bodily fluids
- Items used to distribute or mix hazardous substances

A third-party company routinely collects pharmaceutical garbage. To prepare waste for pickup, place it in bags marked hazardous or biohazard. To store the material until it is picked up, use a bin designed specifically for hazardous waste collection.

Eye Irrigation Station

If medication or other substances are accidently splashed into the eye, utilize the eye irrigation station described below:
- If you are wearing contact lenses, remove them right away.
- Hold the eyes open and arrange the face so that the eyes are appropriately aligned.
- Have someone assist you with turning on the station. Someone else should call for emergency assistance.
- Allow water to constantly flush the eyes until the material has been gone (at least 15 minutes).

Some locations may not have an emergency eyewash station. In this situation, clean the eyes with normal saline and seek emergency medical assistance right away.

Accidental Skin Contact with a Hazardous Substance

Skin contact with a medication or chemical at the drugstore is possible. An inadvertent encounter might result in burns, blisters, rash, hives, irritation, or skin reddening. If exposure occurs, notify a supervisor right once. Remove any contaminated clothing. Apply cool water to the affected area for at least 15 minutes. If the area is painful, apply cool, wet compresses. Cover the burned area with a dry, sterile dressing. If a second or third degree burn has occurred, get medical assistance right away. See page 96 for assessing the severity of burns. The most efficient way to avoid unintended contact with toxic compounds is to always wear personal protective equipment, such as gloves or gowns.

Ingestion of a Hazardous Substance

The treatment for swallowed dangerous substances or poisoning is dictated by the substance.

- Notify your supervisor immediately.
- Identify the material. Locate the substance's Safety Data Sheet and treatment information.
- If necessary, induce vomiting with a product such as ipecac syrup; however, if the chemical is corrosive or the person is unconscious, do not induce vomiting.
- Call for emergency medical assistance immediately.

To avoid accidental consumption, keep food products away from prescription processing facilities at pharmacies and never store foods in refrigerators or freezers used for medicine storage. Furthermore, using a facemask while manufacturing or synthesizing medications will assist in avoiding errors.

Inhalation of a Hazardous Substance

Inhalation of hazardous compounds can occur in the pharmacy while working with powders used for compounding or IV medication preparation. In the event of unintended inhalation, perform these steps:

- Notify a supervisor immediately.
- Evacuate into fresh air.
- Make sure the person who inhaled the toxins is still breathing.
- Call for emergency medical assistance.

When making a powdered product, wear personal protective equipment such a mask to avoid breathing chemicals and hazardous compounds. Although good airflow can prevent a spill from contaminating the entire pharmacy, the area should still be evacuated until it is declared safe.

First, Second, and Third Degree Burns

Burns are classified as first, second, or third degree based on the extent of tissue loss.

- **First-degree burns** are the least severe. The skin may become red, inflamed, and painful, yet the outer layer of skin stays intact. Running cool water over the injured area for 10 to 15 minutes, or using cool compresses, is considered first aid.

- A **second-degree burn** damages the outer layer of skin. Blisters develop, and there may be severe pain and edema. A mild second-degree burn can be treated like a first-degree burn. A significant second-degree burn to the hands, feet, face, or major joint necessitates immediate medical intervention.

- **Third-degree burns** are exceedingly severe. The skin and underlying tissues have been burned completely. The region could be burned or appear white and dry. If you have suffered a third-degree burn, call 911 immediately. If possible, elevate the burned area above the heart and cover with cool, wet, sterile cloths.

Continuing Education

Continuing education publications, papers, and tests are available in a variety of locations. Some pharmaceutical companies host seminars and programs where technicians can obtain continuing education credits. Many pharmaceutical publications have studies that are worth CE credits. Many websites offer CE, including the PTCB website, Powerpak.com, Freece.com, and rxschool.com. Keep track of your CE credits carefully and keep printouts of completed CE credits in case you need to demonstrate compliance. Recertifying takes 20 contact hours, with at least one of them being in pharmaceutical law. Up to ten hours can be earned under the supervision of your pharmacist, but they must be in an area unrelated to your daily responsibilities. Over a two-year period, one college course can be used to earn fifteen continuing education credits.

Updates on Pharmacy Law

The laws governing pharmacies at the state and federal levels are periodically updated. For up-to-date pharmacy legislation knowledge, technicians can refer to the sources listed below:

- The website of the Drug Enforcement Administration can be accessed at www.dea.gov.
- The website for their own state's board of pharmacy
- The website and newsletter of the National Pharmacy Technician Association can be accessed at www.pharmacytechnician.org.
- Pharmacy publications such as Drug Topics, Rx Times, U.S. Pharmacist, and Pharmacy Times

Not only is it vital to stay current with legal changes on a personal and professional level, but one of a certified pharmacy technician's twenty continuing education hours must be legal in order to maintain certification. Examine continuing education resources for courses on pharmaceutical law.

Sterile and Non-Sterile Compounding

Compounded Medication

A compounded drug is a medication that has been made by a pharmacist or technician to meet the doctor's specific dosing recommendations. Compounding may entail changing the dosage form of a medication, such as turning it from powder to cream or capsule to solution. Compounding also includes the creation of tailored injectable medications. Compounding is typically used to address a patient's unique and specific needs, such as individuals who are unable to ingest pills or to offer a dosage that is not otherwise available to a baby. Some compounding, such as adding flavor to a medicine, is done willingly in order to improve adherence.

Compounding

To combine a medicine properly, follow these steps:

- Inputting the prescription into the pharmacy software as directed (some pharmacies may have a separate software system built for compounding prescriptions).
- Setting up the compounding area by doing duties such as cleaning and organizing the compounding paper
- Assembling the correct medications, inert ingredients, and compounding supplies
- Calibrating the equipment
- Performing or double-checking the computations that were provided.
- Compounding medications, using an aseptic method while compounding sterile goods.
- Recording the expiration dates of the compounded medications
- Preparing the order for the pharmacist to review, which includes keeping all equipment packaging as well as the original packaging of the compounded materials.

Compounding Equipment and Supplies

Prior to compounding a cream or ointment, it is necessary to collect the following equipment and supplies:

- Use a Class A prescription balance or analytical balance to weigh the components.
- Weighing papers, for use with the balance
- A spatula is used to move components, such as the base, onto weighing paper or pans.
- If it is necessary to pulverize the particles into a fine powder, employ a mortar and pestle.
- A graduate if liquids will be integrated into the chemical.
- An ointment slab
- The medication to be compounded
- The cream or ointment base
- Wetting agent or levigating agent, if necessary

Equipment Required for Compounding a Sterile Product

In order to produce a sterile product in a controlled environment, it is essential to gather all the required materials prior to commencing the process:

- Personal protective equipment, including gloves, gown, hair bonnet, mask, and foot covers, should be used as necessary.
- It is imperative to perform sterile mixing procedures exclusively under a well sanitized laminar flow hood.
- Vials or ampules of medication to be compounded
- Appropriately sized syringes
- Filter needles if drawing from an ampule

- IV bags or solutions into which the medication will be mixed
- Alcohol for cleaning the hood
- Alcohol wipes are used to sanitize rubber stoppers before inserting a needle.

Checking a Compounded Medication

Prior to the pharmacist's examination of a compounded medication prepared by a technician, the necessary information must be collected:

- The original order and prescription label
- The calculations made to determine the correct dose
- The vials or containers of the medications and solutions used
- When preparing an injectable, the syringe used to remove the drug from the vial is pulled back to the dose utilized.
- If the medication was extracted from an ampule, the packing from the filter needle shows that it was utilized.
- The finished product, free of contamination and particulates

Extemporaneous Compound

An extemporaneous compound, often known as an extemporaneous prescription, is a medication that is prepared by a pharmacist or technician in response to a specific request from a single patient. The compound is produced to meet the prescriber's specific needs for amount, potency, and dosage form, and it contains a pharmaceutical product. Creams, ointments, suspensions, and suppositories are frequently employed extemporaneous compounds. In order to ensure that the mixture has the appropriate dosage of medication and is free from contamination, accurate calculation and meticulous preparation are essential.

Aseptic Technique

The aseptic technique is employed to produce intravenous admixtures and other sterile products. It guarantees the sterility of the products during the preparation process. Inadequate methodology presents a substantial hazard to patients. It is necessary to consistently carry out aseptic procedure within a laminar flow hood. Ensure there is always a space between the HEPA filter and the product being mixed. The airflow guarantees the absence of particulates in the mixture and supplies. Obstructions can be caused by hands, IV bags, and other devices. When extracting product from a syringe or ampule, ensure that you do not contact the plunger except at the back end. Prioritize performing computations before to approaching the hood and ensure that the area remains free of unnecessary items. Prior to entering the neighborhood, ensure that all jewelry is removed from your hands and arms and that they are completely washed. Ensure that you keep your hands within the confines of the hood to the greatest extent possible. If you come into contact with your face, hair, or clothing, it is advisable to wash again. Refrain from engaging in conversation, sneezing, or coughing when working on drug preparation within the enclosed workspace. Prior to puncturing with a needle, sterilize all rubber stoppers with alcohol.

Preparing Sterile Products

When preparing sterile objects, adhere to the following precautions:

- Inspect the medication to verify its current state and confirm that it has not reached its expiration date. A multi-use vial contains preservatives, whereas a single-use vial cannot maintain sterility once it has been pierced and must be discarded, regardless of whether there is any medication left.
- Wash your hands frequently.
- Do not wear jewelry.
- Wear gloves, gown, and bonnet, if required.
- Do not speak or cough into the hood.
- Do not touch the syringe's needle or plunger.
- Wipe rubber stoppers with alcohol before inserting the needle.
- Know aseptic technique, and use it.
- Thoroughly disinfect the preparation area before and after usage.

Medications Considered Sterile Products

The pharmaceuticals listed below are sterile and should be produced as such, using aseptic technique:

- Intravenous medications
- Total parenteral nutrition
- Intramuscular medications
- Ophthalmic solutions and suspensions
- Subcutaneous medications
- Chemotherapy

Sterile products must also be stored in a way that guarantees their sterility. Different drugs have varying storage needs. Consult with your pharmacy manager to learn about the storage protocol at your store. Cover the access port on IV bags to prevent contamination. Foil or plastic coverings are employed for this purpose. Cover this port until the drug is provided to the patient or nurse.

Contamination in Sterile Preparations

Despite best practices and aseptic techniques, contamination can nevertheless occur on occasion. Before distributing sterile medication, check for the following symptoms of contamination:

- Formation of precipitate
- Unidentified objects in the solutions (may indicate that coring has occurred)
- Cloudiness when the solution should be clear
- A change in color that is unanticipated

- A regular needle used to withdraw medication from a glass ampule

- Separation of the ingredients

If the solution cannot be assured to be sterile, show the pharmacist the error-containing solution to help prevent future errors, and then remake the solution.

Proper Hand-Washing Technique

To prepare sterile drugs, hands must be as clean as possible. When preparing medication in a clean environment or beneath a laminar flow hood, employ the hand-washing approach described below:

1. Remove all rings, watches, and other jewelry.

2. Turn on the faucet using your elbow or a paper towel.

3. Wet your hands up to the forearms with warm water.

4. Apply antibacterial soap or a disinfectant solution.

5. Scrub each hand for at least 30 seconds, using the fingers of the other hand.

6. Rinse thoroughly, holding the arms in a downward posture so that the water runs over the fingertips rather than into the garment.

7. Dry your hands using a clean, sterile towel.

8. Turn off the faucet using the sterile towel and discard towel.

Laminar Flow Hood

A laminar flow hood is meant to offer a clean environment for compounding sterile preparations in the pharmacy. Air from the room is pulled through a HEPA filter and blown back toward the user, ensuring that a continual stream of filtered air flows over the items under the hood. Vertical and horizontal are available, as well as customized airflow patterns for specialized applications. To ensure that there are no pollutants, the laminar flow hood must be maintained in accordance with manufacturer requirements and properly cleaned before each usage.

Properly Prepare and Clean the IV Admixture Hood

Cleaning the laminar flow hood requires the appropriate method. This approach includes the following steps:

1. Gather cleaning supplies such as 70% ethanol, sterile gauze, and laboratory-grade wipes.

2. Dress in personal protective equipment including gloves, mask, goggles, foot coverings, and gown.

3. Turn the hood on, and allow the hood to run for five minutes. Remove any items that do not belong in the hood.

4. Spray the disinfectant onto the internal surfaces and clean with sterile wipes in a sweeping back and forth motion. Do not spray disinfectants into the HEPA filter.

5. Allow the hood to air dry.

Total Parenteral Nutrition

Total parenteral nutrition is liquid food given to a patient intravenously.

Parenteral nutrition may be administered for a variety of reasons. For example, the patient may have recently undergone surgery or have a medical condition that prevents him or her from eating orally. Pharmacy technicians are frequently called upon to mix total parenteral nutrition (TPN). TPN contains proteins, carbohydrates, fats, vitamins, and minerals, all of which are required for proper nutrition. To prepare TPN, a pharmacy technician needs complete the following:

- Verify the order, and double check calculations.
- Generate labels, and verify for accuracy.
- Gather ingredients, and mix under a laminar flow hood using a compounder.
- Affix an expiration date of no later than 36 hours.
- Prepare mixture for checking by a pharmacist.

Chemical Incompatibility

Certain drugs are physically and chemically incompatible and should never be combined. Some of the issues that could occur are:

- Formation of precipitates or crystallization
- Formation of gas or other noxious chemical compounds
- The ingredients do not mix to form a solution, for example, one floats on the other or the ingredients congeal

Examples:

- Diazepam dissolves poorly, which can lead to precipitates forming when improperly diluted
- Mixing phenytoin with 5% glucose solution leads to nearly immediate precipitation
- Combining magnesium sulfate and calcium chloride in the same bag will cause a precipitation of calcium sulfate

Medication Safety

Radiopharmaceuticals

A radiopharmaceutical is a drug that a patient consumes to help diagnose or treat disorders such as cancer, colorectal disease, some bone diseases, and others. Radiopharmaceuticals can be administered orally, injected, or instilled into the eye or bladder. Although the agent contains radioactivity, the level is so minimal that it is not detrimental to the body. Some drugs may be used in higher doses for treating a condition. In this case, the impact on the body differs. When a radiopharmaceutical is used to diagnose a problem, the chemical either passes through or is absorbed by the affected organ or system. Radioactivity is detected using specialized equipment, allowing for a diagnosis based on organ or system function.

Chemotherapy

Chemotherapy, often known as antineoplastic medicines, is a class of medications and drug combinations used to treat various types of cancer. The purpose of chemotherapy is to kill rapidly proliferating cells in order to stop and reverse tumor growth. Chemotherapy also kills healthy cells, which causes a variety of negative side effects such as hair loss, nausea, and immunosuppression. Chemotherapy drugs can be administered orally or intravenously. Chemotherapy is frequently used in conjunction with radiation and other treatments to aggressively treat cancer. Some of the several forms of chemotherapy are:

- Alkylating agents like cisplatin and oxaliplatin
- Antimetabolites
- Vinca alkaloids including vincristine and vinblastine
- Taxanes such as paclitaxel and docetaxel

Exposure to Chemotherapy

Working at a pharmacy carries a significant risk of unintentional exposure to chemotherapeutic drugs. This exposure can occur in several ways, including:

- **Inhalation** may occur if a technician breathes in chemotherapy agents that have been aerosolized or distributed as airborne particles.
- **Absorption** may occur if unprotected skin comes into contact with the chemotherapy agent.
- **Ingestion** of the chemotherapy agent can occur from hand to mouth transmission.
- **Injection** can occur due to accidental needle sticks during the preparation of injectable chemotherapy agents.

Chemotherapy medicines can induce a variety of side effects, including rashes, blistering, and irritation. Long-term repercussions could be severe, including miscarriages, birth abnormalities in future children, and cancer.

Chemotherapy Agent's Exposure Prevention

Pharmacies have adopted a number of precautions to protect employees from exposure to chemotherapeutic drugs. Some of these steps are:

- Biological safety cabinets, also known as compounded aseptic containment isolators, are equipped with air filtration systems that supply clean air to the room and safely release the air. These cabinets also feature a glass shield that shields the operator from any potential contact.

- Negatively pressurized clean rooms prevent the spread of contaminated air to adjacent locations.

- The use of personal protective equipment such as gowns, masks, gloves, hair covers, shoe covers, and goggles

- Protocols mandating regular replacement of personal protective equipment to mitigate the risk of contamination

Drug handling procedures encompass the utilization of the negative pressure technique to withdraw pharmaceuticals from vials in order to prevent the dispersion of aerosols and splattering. Additionally, it involves the correct method of extracting medication from ampules and the right disposal of sharps.

Ear and Eye Solutions and Suspensions

Occasionally, doctors may prescribe ocular preparations for use in the ear if the drug and strength are not available in an otic preparation. While this is permissible, it is important to note that otic preparations should not be utilized to fulfill a prescription specifically meant for ocular use. The reason for this is that otic treatments contain preservatives that are not meant to be used in the eyes, which can lead to significant side effects such as burning and itching. When obtaining a drug for use in the eyes or ears, it is crucial to exercise caution and ensure that the correct formulation is chosen. Inform the pharmacist if there is a mistake made by the prescriber. Contacting the prescriber via phone may be required.

Coring the Rubber Stopper

If adequate syringe technique is not employed, there is a risk that a portion of the rubber stopper could break off and become stuck in the hollow needle. This process is commonly referred to as coring, and it possesses the capacity to introduce impurities into the drug, hence posing significant hazards to the patient. If the act of coring remains undetected, and the core is subsequently introduced into the patient's body, it has the potential to result in fatality. In order to avoid coring, it is recommended to insert the needle into the rubber stopper at an angle of 45 to 60 degrees, with the opening oriented upwards and away from the stopper. As the needle is inserted into the stopper, both the pressure and the angle are slightly raised. When inserting the needle through the stopper, it should be positioned at a 90-degree angle or completely vertical.

Counseling by a Pharmacist

Pharmacists must provide counseling to every patient who is given a new prescription. This criterion is mandated by legislation in the majority of states. Counseling serves various objectives:

- It provides a final verification to ensure that the correct patient is receiving the appropriate medication for the correct medical condition.
- The pharmacist can engage in a conversation with the patient about possible adverse reactions and provide guidance on how to handle them, if they arise.
- The feature enables the pharmacist to include and highlight certain directives, such as whether the drug should be consumed with meals or taken at a specific time of day.
- It allows the pharmacist to explain any interactions that may occur.
- It allows the pharmacist to determine the level of health literacy of the patient and adjust instruction accordingly.
- It improves patient compliance.

Common Prescription Errors

Doctors frequently make errors on prescriptions that can be easily checked over the phone. Some of the most prevalent errors are:

- Forgetting to write down the patient's name or writing the incorrect name
- Date errors, such as entering the incorrect date or forgetting to write the date.
- Misspelled medications
- Directions that don't match the medication
- Refills on CII medications
- Forgetting to sign the prescription
- Sloppy handwriting makes it difficult to understand the name of the drug.
- Forgetting to write the quantity or days' supply
- Writing for a dose that doesn't exist
- Simply write "take as directed" ("Take as directed" is not a valid signature.This must be clarified in order to give the exact quantity and days of supply.
- Leaving off the route of administration when more than one is possible

Visual Impairment

Visual impairment can be difficult for people who are receiving drugs or other forms of therapy. Some of the issues that could emerge include:

- Inability to read the directions on the bottle
- Inability to identify the medication based on the size and shape of the pill
- Inability to notice probable pharmaceutical errors (e.g., changes in the hue of a medicine).

Pharmacies can improve the situation in a variety of ways:

- Putting drugs in different sized bottles.
- Providing comprehensive counseling and allowing patients to feel the shape and size of the medication so that they can identify it at home.
- Assisting the patient or caregiver in preparing a Mediset or other method for readily taking drugs that does not require pill bottles (many of which include Braille on the lids).
- Providing handouts in Braille

Syringes

Insulin is dosed in units, hence insulin syringes provide sizes and quantities in units rather than ccs or mLs. Insulin syringes come in a variety of sizes and are fitted with various needle diameters. Needle sizes are measured in both length and gauge. Most insulin syringe needles range from 28 to 31 gauges, with a higher gauge number signifying a finer needle. Patients' personal preferences frequently come into play, as slightly thicker needles are less flexible and can be longer. When purchasing a box of insulin needles, make sure to choose a unit size that is as close to the patient's insulin dose as feasible without going under. If the syringe is too tiny, the patient will need to give two injections. The dosing accuracy deteriorates when the syringe is excessively large.

Signs of Noncompliance in Taking Medications

To work correctly, drugs must be taken exactly as prescribed. According to estimates, at least 10% of all emergency room visits are caused by patients failing to take their medications as prescribed. Every year, many people die as a result of failing to take their prescribed prescriptions in the proper dosages or at all. Patients who are suspected of being noncompliant with their medications should be referred to the pharmacist for further counseling to see what is causing the problem. Some indications that identify noncompliant patients are:

- Consistently late refills
- Questions about splitting pills when the dose doesn't require it
- Dropping off multiple prescriptions but only filling one
- Phone calls from the doctor about missed appointments

Missed Dose

Always send patients who have missed a dosage or have any questions regarding their medicine to a pharmacist for advice. What the patient should do is mostly dependent on which medication was missed. Most prescriptions require the patient to take the missed dose as soon as they notice it, or, if the next dose is approaching, to forego the missed dose and take the following dose as planned. Other drugs need the patient to take a double dose the following day. However, some medications must be taken exactly as prescribed and should be completely avoided if missed.

Drug Stability

A variety of factors contribute to drug stability. Some drugs degrade faster when exposed to light (they must be stored in opaque or darkly tinted bottles), others when exposed to heat (they must be refrigerated), and still others when exposed to oxygen (their expiration date changes once opened).As a result, medications that are distributed must have an expiration date on the bottle no later than one year after the dispensing date. Medications that have been mixed frequently have a post-mixing expiration period printed on the bottle (for example, 10 days after mixing), which should be used to establish the expiry date. When nitroglycerin tablets are opened, they decay, so pharmacists should advise patients on their expiration dates.

Epidural Administration vs. Intravenous Administration

When preparing drugs for epidural injection, it is critical that they include no preservatives. Medications for epidural administration must be carefully marked to avoid confusion and unintentional administration of intravenous medications. Preservative-containing medications administered by epidural pose a high risk of neurotoxicity and adverse effects, such as epidural tissue destruction and neurological symptoms. Preservative-free drugs and those containing preservatives should be kept separate in the pharmacy to avoid errors. To avoid mix-ups, technicians doing admixture should prepare drugs for intravenous and epidural use in different batches.

Extravasation

Extravasation occurs when drugs intended for intravenous delivery are given into tissue surrounding the location rather than the vein. This can happen in a variety of ways:

- Leakage caused by damaged veins. This happens on occasion in the elderly and in those with compromised veins.
- Leaking from a hole in the vein that was created by a previous injection
- Improper technique when placing the infusion

Extravasation is a severe adverse occurrence that can cause a variety of side effects, including tissue necrosis. While every drug might provide side effects, extravasation with chemotherapy is especially troubling.

Health Literacy

Health literacy refers to a person's ability to understand and make healthcare decisions for themselves. Health literacy encompasses a wide range of abilities, from a complete lack of understanding, which leads to medication errors, missed appointments, and noncompliance, to a thorough understanding of how insurance companies operate, as well as a good understanding of how multiple systems in the body work. Individuals with inadequate health literacy may require additional counseling and assistance to receive appropriate medical care. Being aware of your patients' potential health literacy and referring those who may be less health literate to the pharmacist for additional counseling is a beneficial service to them.

Low Health Literacy

Some of the population categories who are likely to have inadequate health literacy and require further assistance are:

- The elderly
- Immigrants

- Minorities
- People with lower income

While it is necessary to identify people with inadequate health literacy so that they can receive additional counseling, it is also crucial to avoid using stereotypes that may be offensive. An elderly patient, such as a retired doctor, may feel upset if they are treated as if they are unaware of how their drug works. Listen carefully to your patients' words, including the questions they ask and the worries they express, to identify those with inadequate health literacy.

Additional Pharmacist Counseling

While certain groups of people are more likely to have low health literacy, not all of them have issues. It is critical to identify individuals who face problems while without disparaging those who do not. Some symptoms that a patient may need additional support include:

- A patient who cannot identify the condition for which they have been prescribed the drug.
- A patient who nods his or her head when asked a question but does not answer
- A patient who agrees to everything but doesn't ask informed questions
- A patient who fills out an intake form incorrectly or leaves big parts blank.
- Statements such as "I will read this later" or "I forgot my glasses"

Communication with Patients

As a pharmacy technician, you may improve treatment for persons with limited health literacy by doing the following:

- Identifying people who appear to have low health literacy and informing the pharmacist
- Listening to the concerns patients express and bringing the pharmacist over to help answer the patient's questions
- Speaking simply and without using medical jargon (for example, referring to a medication as a "blood pressure pill" instead of "antihypertensive")
- Using short sentences
- Selecting appropriate auxiliary labels
- Asking the patient questions to confirm understanding
- Maintain a friendly and inviting demeanor to make the patient feel more comfortable.

Patient Counseling

The pharmacist is the only one who should provide patient counseling. When under the supervision of a preceptor, a pharmacy intern may be permitted to counsel. Every patient must have access to counseling. The pharmacist's goal is to ensure that the patient knows the directions, adverse effects, and other critical information concerning the medicine. During a counseling session, more information may be acquired, such as the ailment the medicine is intended to treat and any other medications the patient is taking. These sessions are critical for ensuring that the patient takes the medication appropriately, improving compliance, and helping the patient's condition improve.

Counseling Refusal

Patients may refuse counseling if the medicine is a refill or if the patient has been taking the medication for some time (but pharmacist counseling should still be offered if the patient has any questions or concerns). If a patient declines counseling, they must give a record with their signature. This record may be saved electronically or as a file. The individual providing therapy should never employ a voice or tone that suggests that counseling the patient would be bothersome or inconvenient. The ultimate goal is to increase patient safety, which can be partially accomplished by advising all patients.

Unnecessary or Expired Medications

When prescriptions that are no longer needed or that have expired are kept about the house, the following problems may arise:

- Diversion from family members or guests in the household
- Drugs may be retrieved from the trash and sold or abused
- Drugs may be found by children and ingested, leading to accidental poisonings, especially if the medications are not stored in their original containers with child-resistant caps
- Drugs may be disposed of improperly, leading to further abuse or damage to the environment
- Medications taken after the expiration date may be less effective or potentially hazardous.

Child Resistant Caps

Child resistant caps, often known as child resistant packaging, are designed to prevent accidents and deaths caused by children using drugs. To open the bottles, the lids use a device that demands knowledge of the technique as well as manual dexterity. Some caps need to be compressed or forced downward to open, while others need to have their lines matched. Every prescription must be dispensed with child-resistant caps. The patient has the option to waive this obligation, usually by signing a waiver that releases the pharmacy from duty. Local laws and procedures governing how this is handled will differ.

Child Resistant Verses Childproof Caps

When discussing packaging designed to prevent children from opening it, the recommended word is "child resistant." It is referred to in this manner to help instill the belief that no package will ever be completely childproof. Even child-resistant containers and bottles should be kept out of children's reach to avoid potentially fatal poisonings and overdoses. Children have been known to learn how to open child-resistant caps and containers. Packaging should never be viewed as the only line of defense.

Tetracycline

Tetracycline is an exception to the rule of never using a drug after it has expired. Tetracycline medications, such as minocycline, become harmful after their expiration date.

Chemicals in the capsules degrade and can cause kidney harm if consumed after the expiration date. If a course of tetracycline is ended before completion as directed by a doctor, the remaining drug should be disposed of appropriately. Do not discontinue taking antibiotics without consulting a doctor or pharmacist. Discontinuing antibiotics early may result in a recurrence of the infection and adds to the spread of drug-resistant bacteria.

Phone Calls

As a technician, it's crucial to understand which phone calls are within their scope of competence and which should be directed to a pharmacist. The technician can handle the following calls:

- General store information queries
- Requests for refills
- Questions regarding quantities of refills left
- Pricing questions
- Questions regarding insurance

Any phone calls requiring specialized expertise or professional guidance must be directed to the pharmacist. This includes:

- Questions about the actions of medications
- Questions about interactions
- Recommendations for medications or other treatment
- New prescriptions calls from doctors
- Any other questions requiring medical advice

Pharmacy Quality Assurance

Improve Quality Control and Prevent Mistakes

Preventing mistakes is a primary priority for every pharmacy. Typical quality control measures are:

- Counseling every patient on the proper use of the medication
- Avoiding abbreviations and medical jargon
- Identifying "sound-alike" medications (for example, Celebrex and Celexa, Lamictal and Lamisil) and marking them in the pharmacy to raise awareness.
- Identifying and marking "high alert" drugs within the pharmacy, such as warfarin.
- Using computer software to uncover probable interactions and therapeutic duplicates (do not skip checks)
- Taking the time to properly check and double-check drugs and not allow oneself to be rushed.
- Reporting any errors appropriately to identify system failures and improve the process
- Keeping appropriate levels of trained staff in the pharmacy at all times

Calibration

Calibration is necessary for many pharmaceutical items to maintain patient safety, medicine integrity, and prevent erroneous dosing. The following are examples of pharmacy equipment that should be maintained and calibrated on a regular basis:

- Scales that are used to count medications
- Scales used to weigh ingredients for compounding
- Thermometers in the refrigerator, freezer, and general pharmacy space
- Air samplers in clean rooms
- Machinery used to compound medications

Always follow the manufacturer's instructions when calibrating equipment.

Infection Control

Infection control is the process of implementing procedures inside a healthcare facility to avoid the spread of communicable diseases. The policies aid in preventing transmission from employee to employee, employee to patient, patient to employee, and patient to patient. Most facilities have a section dedicated solely to creating and monitoring quality control procedures and rules inside the system to verify their effectiveness. Healthcare-related infections are a major issue in hospitals, especially because hospital-acquired illnesses might be more deadly than infections obtained outside. Nosocomial infections are another term for healthcare-associated infections.

Hospital Infection Control Officer

An infection control officer in a hospital or other healthcare facility is often a doctor, registered nurse, or epidemiologist who specializes in disease prevention. The purpose of this post is to prevent the spread of contagious diseases in hospitals. The officer accomplishes this purpose by developing rules and practices throughout the hospital, training staff on the policies, and monitoring staff for compliance. Infection control officers might operate independently or as part of a larger infection control team. Large hospitals typically have infection control teams dedicated to preventing infections in all departments, including pharmacy.

Infection Control Procedures

Infection control practices and policies commonly encountered in healthcare settings include:

- Teaching good hand washing techniques and providing various stations to facilitate and encourage frequent hand cleaning.
- Aseptic medication preparation and administration
- Providing personal protective equipment, including masks, gloves, gowns, and more
- Ensuring appropriate sterilization of equipment by using alcohol and other disinfectants or autoclaves
- Tracking vaccination records of employees
- Making seasonal vaccinations easily accessible
- Requiring regular testing for communicable diseases such as TB
- Writing and posting a plan for bloodborne pathogen exposure
- Policies for management of infectious waste
- Investigating any outbreaks that may occur
- Giving preventative treatment in the event of an accidental exposure

Sharps

A sharp is a medical equipment that has the capacity to break the skin and pose a risk of harm and bloodborne disease transmission. Sharps most commonly relate to injection needles, but they can also refer to razor blades, broken glass, scalpels, and other similar instruments. Sharps must be disposed of properly to avoid damage, especially to staff who handle rubbish. Personal protective equipment may not be sufficient to avoid injuries from sharps because needles and other sharps can often cut through medical gloves. The best way to avoid injury from sharps is by careful handling and correct disposal.

Recapping Needles

In most cases, needles should not be recapped. This method frequently results in injuries, such as sticks and inadvertent injections of drugs. If a needle needs to be recapped, never recap it with one hand while holding the cap in the other. Either use tongs to hold the cap or place it on a flat surface and insert the needle. Always dispose of needles in the approved sharps disposal container. Any needle stick or injury should be reported immediately to your supervisor and the infection control officer.

Disposal of Sharps

Sharps should always be disposed of in the proper manner. Special containers designed to hold spent sharps are available for purchase at pharmacies and medical supply stores in a variety of sizes. Containers can be disposed off at specified disposal locations, such as hospitals, doctors' offices, and pharmacies. There are also products available that will degrade needles and make them safe for disposal. Examples include devices that melt or sever the needle, making it harmless. Each state has rules governing the proper disposal of sharps, therefore it is critical to check local laws to ensure that you are following them.

Good customer service

Patients that visit a pharmacy for services are sick, in pain, or have another issue or worry. Providing outstanding customer service and making them feel more at ease will go a long way toward alleviating their condition. Although patients may appear irritated or short-tempered, the person servicing them must realize that a customer's irritation or anger is usually not directed at them.

Long lines and waits, troubles with insurance companies, and the odd need to clarify a prescription with the physician can all add to the frustration of pharmacy visits. Remaining calm and resolving events as they arise will go a long way toward improving the customer's overall pharmacy experience.

Ensuring Good Customer Service

Some ways to ensure good customer service in a pharmacy:

- Provide special aid to anyone who appears to be sick or in pain. Provide a drink or a place to sit while they wait.
- Never dispute with a consumer. Always have a pleasant and calm demeanor. If a consumer becomes abusive, contact a pharmacist or other supervisor for help.
- Avoid employing slang when assisting elderly patients. Many people may misunderstand or be offended by what you're saying.
- Offer to assist anyone who looks like he or she needs help.
- Maintain a neutral expression and demeanor, regardless of whether the drug is being delivered or picked up. Never let personal feelings or judgment appear.
- Give the patient your complete attention. Do not type or answer the phone while aiding a customer.
- If you do not know the answer to a question, find someone who does.

Better Customer Service to Senior Citizens

Many elderly people will visit pharmacies. Here are some ways a pharmacy technician might give superior customer service to senior citizens:

- Speak slowly and enunciate, as they may be hard of hearing.
- Use plain language and avoid slang and medical jargon.
- Provide a place for them to sit while waiting.
- Listen carefully when they are speaking.
- Many senior citizens may no longer drive and may be waiting for a ride. Try to get their prescription ready quickly.
- Check profiles carefully for polypharmacy and potential interactions. Point these out to the pharmacist for additional counseling opportunities.

Pharmacy Chain of Command

In a typical retail pharmacy situation, particularly in a chain shop, the chain of command is as follows:

1. Pharmacy clerk or assistant
2. Pharmacy technician (uncertified)
3. Pharmacy technician (certified)
4. Lead technician
5. Pharmacy intern
6. Pharmacist
7. Pharmacy supervisor
8. District pharmacy supervisor
9. Regional pharmacy supervisor

When a problem emerges, it is critical to move up the chain of command. Attempt to tackle problems locally (inside the location) first. If the situation cannot be resolved or if it is with the person directly above you in the chain of command, you may need to work your way up. Not every stage in the chain will always be there.

Hospital Pharmacy Chain of Command

In a normal hospital pharmacy context, chain of command can be difficult to determine, especially if the pharmacy has many sites or satellites. A technician operating in an oncology satellite may report to a different supervisor than a technician working at the main filling station. Generally, the chain of command has this structure:

1. Pharmacy clerk or assistant
2. Pharmacy technician
3. Certified pharmacy technician
4. Lead technician (may be more than one)
5. Pharmacy intern
6. Pharmacist
7. Pharmacy supervisor (may be more than one)
8. Director of pharmacy staff

It is critical to understand the chain of command for your specific organization, as well as any modifications based on your position within it.

Workflow

Workflow is a method of organizing job responsibilities such that each stage in the process flows easily into the next, increasing work efficiency and saving time and energy. Every pharmacy will have their own method of organizing work to ensure that it runs well, and good pharmacies will be continuously searching for ways to update and improve their workflow. Ideally, each phase should seamlessly transition to the next, allowing for immediate progress. Learning the pharmacy's workflow and your role within it is the first step toward completing your obligations as needed and preventing work from bottlenecking or backing up.

Scheduling

The scheduling may be done by the supervising pharmacist or delegated to a technician or another staff member. Many significant considerations must be made when scheduling pharmacy workers. The most fundamental element of scheduling is to ensure that there are enough staff available to perform the work quickly and efficiently while staying within budget. This means that employees must arrive on time for their assigned shifts and stay until the end of the shift. Failure to show up for a shift places an additional load on other employees and can drastically disrupt workflow.

Cross Training

In most pharmacies, pharmacy technicians are responsible for a variety of activities. While retail pharmacies typically require pharmacy technicians to handle all necessary activities, technicians in a hospital setting are frequently taught in one area until they have mastered those skills, ensuring that jobs are completed as efficiently as possible. However, having technicians educated to operate in a variety of areas benefits the pharmacy. This opens up more scheduling alternatives and increases flexibility inside the pharmacy. Requesting cross-training in other departments of the pharmacy will boost your worth as an employee while also allowing you to expand your knowledge and experiences.

Multitasking

Multitasking is the ability to accomplish multiple tasks at the same time, such as typing a prescription while answering a phone call or greeting a customer while ringing out another. While multitasking allows you to complete more tasks, it can also have major drawbacks. When two tasks requiring accuracy are completed concurrently, each is likely to suffer. Counting medicine, compounding drugs, IV admixture, and order entry are all duties that require your whole attention. It is time-consuming to redo work that has been completed wrongly. Furthermore, pursuing another work while catering to a customer may make the consumer feel unimportant or unworthy of your entire attention, resulting in lost revenue. One of the rare exceptions is to acknowledge newly arrived customers. Interrupt your work, inform the customer that you will be with them shortly, and then return to your project with double-checked correctness.

First Aid Kit

First aid kits are essential items that should always be stocked in the pharmacy. The Red Cross recommends that every first aid kit include the following items:

- Absorbent compresses
- Adhesive bandages
- Adhesive cloth tape
- Antibiotic ointment
- Antiseptic wipes
- Aspirin
- Hydrocortisone ointment
- Instant cold compresses
- Instruction booklet
- Non-latex gloves
- Roller bandages
- Sterile gauze pads
- Thermometer
- Triangular bandages
- Tweezers

First aid kits can be purchased as a unit or assembled independently. When checking expiration dates on the rest of the pharmacy inventory, make sure to check the first aid kit as well. It may be useful to create a label with the earliest expiration date in the kit so that it can be replaced as needed.

Fire Extinguisher

Understand the locations of all fire extinguishers in the pharmacy. Read the instructions carefully and understand how to use the extinguisher before an emergency strikes. The acronym PASS identifies the procedures for utilizing a fire extinguisher.

- Pull the pin on top of the extinguisher to unlock it.
- Aim the extinguisher's nozzle at the base of the flames. This will reduce the fuel and prevent the fire from spreading.
- Squeeze the lever in a slow and controlled motion.
- Sweep side to side. Begin at a safe distance then draw in closer as the fire fades.

Accidental Finger Stick

When working with needles, finger sticks are a significant risk. If you accidentally stick your finger while preparing medications, you risk injecting yourself with the medication.

For some drugs, this could be quite harmful. If a finger stick happens, notify your supervisor right away and follow these steps:

- Encourage bleeding to help flush out the injected medication.
- Wash the area with soap and water.
- Follow your organization's medical treatment policy. You may also need a tetanus vaccine.

If you are mistakenly stuck with a needle used on a patient, follow the same procedure, but the HIV status of the individual who was previously stuck with the needle must be determined. Please notify your infection control supervisor immediately. You will most likely need to start post-exposure prophylaxis.

Post-Exposure Prophylaxis

Post-exposure prophylaxis (PEP) is treatment and medicine given to someone after probable HIV exposure with the purpose of reducing the risk of contracting HIV. Ideally, treatment should begin within an hour of exposure. The protocol usually involves an anti-retroviral medication regimen as well as follow-up testing and treatment. Although the risk of transmission from a needle stick or other sharps contact is less than 1%, infection control should be alerted right after so that the occurrence may be documented and treatment can begin. While PEP can help prevent transmission, it is preferable to use safe needle handling procedures to avoid needle sticks and other forms of inadvertent exposure altogether.

Good Personal Hygiene

Personal cleanliness is critical in every aspect of healthcare, including pharmacy. When visiting a healthcare facility, keep your clothes clean and stain-free, your hair washed and pulled back, your facial hair neatly trimmed (check your location's policies as some may not allow facial hair), and your hands clean. You are not only representing your organization to clients and patients who may be put off by a cluttered appearance, but you are also handling prescriptions and medical equipment. Dirty hands can contaminate medication and equipment. Loose hair can get into drugs or brush equipment. Clean clothes reduce the spread of pathogens and are an important infection control tool.

Healthy Pharmacy Technician

If you are unwell with a viral or bacterial infection, you should not report to work. You risk not only making the rest of your coworkers sick, but also infecting patients who may have compromised immune systems as a result of their own health conditions or therapy. This is particularly important for pharmacy technicians preparing chemotherapy or working in oncology satellites. A technician can come to work with a minor cold, but they must wear a mask and avoid contact with patients who have weaker immune systems. If you are not feeling well, notify your supervisor.

Evaluate Employees

Typically, employees are assessed every six months or annually. Evaluations are provided through a variety of techniques, including:

- Supervisor evaluations, in which the supervisor grades the employee in a number of different categories and specifies areas in which the person succeeds and areas that may require development.
- Peer evaluations, in which the coworkers of the employee are asked to rate him or her
- Self-evaluations, in which employees are asked to appraise themselves, noting both their strengths and areas where they may need to improve.

Depending on the position, both observational and numerical data may be employed. Accuracy, efficiency, competence, and customer service abilities are common criteria for ranking pharmacy technicians.

Self-Evaluations vs. Peer Evaluations

Peer evaluations are useful for evaluating employees since peers may often reveal qualities and weaknesses that a supervisor may not see. Self-evaluations are frequently regarded the most difficult sort of assessment. Employees are asked to define their own strengths and to identify areas for growth. Instead than focusing solely on your strengths, it's important to mention areas where you feel you may improve. This allows you to interact with your employer and ask for help. Employers value employees who take responsibility for their own development and training.

Medication Order Entry and Fill Process

Ways a Pharmacy Receives a Valid Prescription

A prescription may be:

- Brought in by a patient or a patient's representative
- Phoned in by a doctor or a doctor's representative
- Faxed
- Transmitted electronically
- Transferred between pharmacies, via pharmacist-to-pharmacist communication
- Refills can be requested directly by the patient or their agent, through the pharmacy's refill request system, or by phone.

Prescriptions may also be accepted after correcting ambiguous information. Limitations include: a) a CII drug cannot be sent via fax or electronic transfer (though this is permitted in some circumstances), and b) a pharmacist must check the accuracy of a prescription received by phone or electronically.

Processing a Patient's Prescription

When a prescription arrives at the pharmacy, it is processed as follows:

- The prescription and its associated information are entered into the patient's profile.
- The appropriate product is selected for filling the prescriptions.
- The product required to fill the prescriptions is obtained from stock.
- The correct quantity is calculated and dispensed.
- The finished product is appropriately packaged.
- The prescription label and any additional labels are fastened to the container.
- Any necessary patient information materials are collected and assembled.
- The prescription is verified for accuracy (for example, by checking the NDC number).
- Medication and prescription are prepared for final check.

All information is checked by a tech or a pharmacist according to the relevant law.

Medication Calculation

To accurately determine the quantity of a medication, the days' supply and dosing instructions are required. If both of these are available, multiply the days' supply by the number of doses needed each day. For example, if the prescription instructs the patient to take the drug three times each day for seven days, the dose supplied would be 21.

To calculate the days' supply of a medication, the number of doses to be administered and the dosing instructions must be provided. If both options are available, divide the total number of doses to be dispensed by the number of doses each day. For instance, if a patient takes two pills per day, the total number of administered doses is 28, resulting in a 14-day supply.

Prescription Label Information

The following information must be mentioned on the prescription label.

- Dispensing pharmacy's name, address, and telephone number
- Directions for use
- Dispensing pharmacist's name or initials
- The prescription serial number
- The medication's name
- The date of the fill or refill
- The medication's strength
- Prescriber's name
- Quantity of medication dispensed
- Patient's name

Most pharmacies utilize software to automatically generate prescription labels that include all of this information. However, in the event of a software or power failure, the information should be handwritten on the label. Technicians should understand the information that must be included.

Auxiliary Label

The auxiliary label offers additional information regarding the drug that is not included on the prescription label, such as cautions and qualifications. Common supplementary labels include instructions for storage, unconventional routes of administration, food or water requirements, and cautions about potentially harmful side effects. It is usually believed that no more than three auxiliary labels should be placed on the bottle, but the number of labels may be limited by the bottle's size. Auxiliary labels must be placed so that they do not obscure any of the necessary information on the prescription labels. Some of the most prevalent auxiliary labels are:

- Do not crush
- Do not drink alcoholic beverages while taking this medication
- May cause drowsiness
- Store in refrigerator
- Take with food

- Medication should be taken with water
- For the nose
- For the ears

Informational Products

A variety of informational materials and pamphlets may be necessary to accompany the prescription when it is presented to the patient. Some pharmaceuticals are legally required to provide "black box warning" information sheets that explain potentially harmful side effects. Each prescription should be accompanied by HIPAA material. Each new prescription must include printed information about the medication, including potential side effects and administration instructions. These patient handouts are not intended to replace pharmacist-provided counseling.

Tech Check Tech

In rare cases, pharmacy technicians are permitted to review another technician's work. Laws enabling this differ by state. In many circumstances, technicians permitted to inspect other technicians have received further training on the process. In other circumstances, technicians check fills before a pharmacist conducts a final check. Some refill centers permit the practice since a pharmacist has previously reviewed the initial prescription. "Tech check tech" programs are not commonly employed in community pharmacies, but can be found in hospital pharmacies, long-term care pharmacies, and other institutional settings.

V Solution Flow Rate Calculation

The flow rate of IV solutions, sometimes known as the drip rate, is calculated in milliliters per hour. To calculate the mL/hr. for any solution, you must first know the total volume of the bag to be infused (for example, 1000 mL) as well as the duration of the infusion (for example, 8 hours). In this example, divide the bag's total mL by the number of hours to get a flow rate of 125 mL/hr.

If the solution is to be infused for less than an hour, divide the mL by the number of minutes and multiply by 60.For example, if a 150 mL piggyback is to be infused for 30 minutes, divide it by 30 to get 5.Multiply 5 by 60 to get 300.The flow rate is 300 mL/hour.

Distributing Medication

When distributing medications to a patient in the community setting, the following processes must be followed:

- Store the medication properly prior to distribution.
- Make sure that all supplemental information is prepared.
- If you do not know the patient, check their identify by seeking identification or asking them to confirm their birthdate or residence. Follow your location's protocol.
- If a patient's representative is picking up the drug, it may be important to affirm that this individual is authorized to do so. Again, adhere to your location's process.
- Deliver the medication to the patient or patient's representative.
- Provide pharmacist counseling to the patient.

- Record the distribution as legally required.

Reconstituting Powder for Oral Suspension

Many drugs are in powder form and must be reconstituted to generate an oral solution. These medications should be reconstituted at the time of purchase, when the consumer is present to collect them. Early reconstitution can cause the drug to expire prematurely. Patients should not reconstitute powders since wrong reconstitution could result in erroneous dose. Additionally, using tap water to reconstitute may add pollutants. Pharmacies have a gadget that reconstitutes drugs with sterile water. Some use automated methods, while others rely on gravity. Check the amount of water required to reconstitute the drug as indicated on the label. Enter this number into the automated system or fill the reservoir to the exact amount. Fill the bottle, stopping halfway through to shake and mix (many automated systems allow for a mix while delivering water). Before giving the drug, thoroughly shake the product to verify that it has been completely blended.

Dispensing Investigational Drugs

Some pharmacies, particularly those located in research and university hospitals, sell investigational medications used in research. The majority of the regulations and protocols for dispensing investigational medications are similar to those for dealing with any prescription drug. The medicine requires doctor's orders and a valid documented prescription. Other needs that are particular for experimental medications include:

- Verification of research or study protocol
- Verification of informed consent from the patient
- Record keeping specific to the study medication
- On-site preparation and storage of the product
- Unique disposal requirements for the product

Automatic Stop Order

Automatic stop orders are safety precautions that prevent drugs from being used for an extended period of time or beyond what is considered safe. Many hospitals use automatic cease orders for drugs such short-term opioids, antibiotics, and ketorolac. Some systems may automatically cancel medicine prescriptions if the patient is transported to or from a different level of care, such as the critical care unit or surgery. The doctor must reassess and rewrite the drug orders. Individual pharmacies' regulations regarding automatic stop orders may vary. Check to see what your pharmacy's protocol is.

Patient Controlled Analgesic

A patient-controlled analgesic, or PCA, is a drug that is produced and given using a preprogrammed infusion pump. It enables the patient to deliver a predetermined quantity of intravenous pain medicine as needed for comfort and pain control, while limiting the amount that can be administered to avoid overdose. PCA devices are frequently used after surgery or childbirth, when patients are awake enough to press the handheld button. Only the patient to whom the PCA device is attached may press the button to distribute the medication. Family members, friends, and other visitors may not dispense the drug, even if they believe they are assisting the patient. If the patient is not attentive enough to distribute medication, he or she is not a suitable candidate for a PCA.

Tinted Prescription Bottles

Medicine storage bottles in pharmacies are typically opaque. Medications are administered in bottles that are either opaque or colored. Many drugs contain ingredients that are sensitive to light. Excessive exposure to light causes the drug to deteriorate, reducing its potency and lifetime. This is known as a photochemical reaction. While amber is perhaps the most prevalent prescription bottle color, additional options include dark brown, dark green, and red. To safeguard the drug's integrity, patients should use a tinted Mediset or store it in a dark cupboard while using a medication tracking system.

Prepackaged Medication

Many pharmacies, particularly hospital or clinic pharmacies, buy medication in bulk and prepackage it into bottles in regularly used quantities for rapid distribution. This procedure saves the pharmacy money because the substance can be purchased in bulk. It also saves time by eliminating the need to count out typical doses many times. A pharmacist checks the prepacking, so when it comes time to distribute, the pharmacist simply needs to ensure that the pre-packed medication contains the proper amount and quantity indicated for the patient. Antibiotics and nonsteroidal anti-inflammatory drugs are two common pharmaceuticals for prepackaging.

Robotics

Robotics and automated dispensing systems are increasingly employed in high-volume pharmacies to increase accuracy, save manual labor, reduce inventory, and eliminate the need for checking. McKesson's Robot-Rx and ScriptPro's Compact Robotic System (or CRS) are two examples of current robotics applications. Robotics in pharmacy aim to free up pharmacists and technicians from repetitive chores, allowing them to focus on patient care. Large central fill facilities that dispense thousands of prescriptions each day are more likely to use robotic dispensers.

The Baker Cell

McKesson Automation manufactures the Baker Cell device. When a prescription is typed into the interface, the information is communicated to the device, which dispenses the appropriate number of pills. The system's goal is to reduce time spent delivering medication. A Baker Cell can count as much as 600 tablets per minute. The cell allows the pharmacy to boost the volume of orders dispensed while also freeing up staff time for other operations. The system can be modified and customized to meet almost any pharmacy setting.

Automated TPN Compounding Equipment

Total parental nutrition compounding is frequently done in pharmacies. Because there are so many components involved in TPN preparation, each of which must be exactly accurate, many pharmacies use automated TPN equipment to limit the risk of errors and promote patient safety. These systems allow a pharmacist or technician to enter an order into a computer, which calculates the appropriate dose for dispensing. To maintain sterility and prevent contamination, the procedure requires monitoring and setup. Some popular automated TPN systems that a technician may encounter include Abbot's Nutramix, Baxa's Exacta Mix, and Secure's AutoComp.

Pyxis

Pyxis is a renowned brand of automated dispensing software that is utilized in hospitals and other medical facilities across the country. The systems are easily customizable and can range from a single tiny cabinet to a more comprehensive system that includes refrigeration and automated drawers. Pyxis monitors inventory in its system and generates reports that technicians can use to refill as needed. Pyxis can also be coupled with pharmacy software, allowing nurses to access just medications expressly prescribed for a patient while pharmacists and doctors can track prescriptions dispensed. Pyxis systems are extremely secure, with password protection and additional security features like as fingerprint scanning to assure the safety and security of the pharmaceuticals contained within.

Infusion Pump

Infusion pumps are programmable devices that regulate the flow rate of various types of infusions. The most typical application is intravenous infusion, but subcutaneous and epidural infusions can also be routed via a pump. Infusion pumps can be configured to administer irregular doses of medication or to offer continuous infusion. Infusion pumps can also be set to provide patient-controlled analgesia. There are two types of infusion pumps: large volume pumps for infusing fluids like complete parenteral nutrition, and tiny volume pumps for administering insulin.

Total Parenteral Nutrition Solutions

Most complete parenteral solutions adhere to a specified formula. Batching orders simplifies the process for both prescribers and those processing them. TPN solutions are classified into two types: 2-in-1 solutions (amino acid and dextrose) and 3-in-1 solutions (amino acid, dextrose, and fat).Other typical components of TPN solutions are:

- Fluid, often in the form of water
- Electrolytes, which include sodium, calcium, magnesium, potassium, and phosphate
- Vitamins, including A, B-complex, C, D, and folic acid
- Minerals, such as copper, chromium, manganese, and zinc.

Pharmacy Inventory Management

Generic Medication

A generic drug is a pharmaceutical produced by a separate company that matches the brand-name medication in the following areas:

- Active ingredient
- Route of administration
- Dosage form
- Intended use
- Strength Quality and performance characteristics

The drug's generic name is the medication's nonproprietary name. The Food and Drug Administration regulates generic medications, and the maker must demonstrate that they are equal to their brand-name counterpart within an allowed bioequivalent range. If the generic name is specified on the prescription, it might be used instead of the brand name. It can also be substituted if the physician has marked the prescription "substitution permitted" or neglected to label it "dispense as written."

Therapeutic Substitution

A therapeutic substitute is a drug that differs from the one originally prescribed. Unlike generic substitutions, the medication may differ in dosage form, manner of administration, or performance characteristics. Therapeutic substitution can be done for a variety of reasons. The prescriber is generally consulted, however this is not always essential under certain conditions. The most common grounds for therapeutic substitution are:

- The third-party payer does not cover the prescribed medication.
- The prescribed medication is too expensive.
- The prescribed medication is unavailable.
- The prescribed medication is less convenient.

NDC Number

The National Drug Code number (NDC number) is a ten-digit identifier that distinguishes each individual drug suitable for human use. The Drug Listing Act of 1972 introduced NDC numbers. Each part of the 10-digit code represents an aspect of the medication:

- The first part, the labeler code, identifies the medication's maker.

- The second part is the product code, which defines the medication's strength and dosing form.
- The package code is the third segment and identifies the quantity and packaging type of the medication.

If a product is no longer in production, its NDC number cannot be redistributed. The NDC number uniquely identifies each product, so technicians and pharmacists can utilize it to improve patient safety by comparing the code on the package to the code on the prescription to ensure that the patient is receiving the correct drug.

Dispense as Written

When prescribing a drug, the doctor can instruct the pharmacy to dispense it as written. When a prescription is to be dispensed as written, the pharmacist must fill it with the exact medication indicated, even if a generic version is available. This could happen for a number of reasons:

- The patient may prefer the brand name medication.
- The prescriber may prefer the brand name medication.
- The patient may have an allergy to one of the inactive ingredients in the generic.

If the medication is not available in the form specified in the prescription, the pharmacy must obtain approval from the prescriber before making any changes to the prescription.

Refrigerated Medications Storage

Some drugs must be stored under refrigeration to maintain their efficacy. Every pharmacy must have a dedicated refrigerator on site to store drugs that require refrigeration. Other things, including food for consumption, should not be stored in this refrigerator. Refrigerator temperatures should range from 2 to 8 degrees Celsius (36-46 degrees Fahrenheit).The temperature should be monitored and reported on a regular basis to ensure that pharmaceuticals are stored at the proper temperature. Biological drugs like insulin, several vaccines, and certain suppositories are examples of common pharmaceuticals that must be refrigerated.

Unit Dose

Medication is frequently packaged in unit doses at hospital and long-term care pharmacies. Unit dosage drugs have three unique functions:

1. They prevent dosing errors.

2. They prevent drug diversion.

3. They save time during drug distribution.

Unit dose packaging is subject to the same restrictions as other drug products. The package must include the patient's name, pharmacy name, address, and phone number, the name of the medication, strength, and instructions for use, the expiration date, and the quantity contained in the container. When medications are unit dosed, their expiration date must be calculated based on the date they were packaged and cannot be more than six months, even if the bulk container indicates a later date.

Proper Storage Conditions

Medications that do not require refrigeration or other special handling conditions should be kept at room temperature, which is defined as between 68 and 77 degrees Fahrenheit, with only minor deviations. However, the average temperature should not exceed 77 degrees. To maintain this temperature, pharmacies should have operating heaters and air conditioners as needed dependent on the local weather. A diary should be kept at the pharmacy to record daily temperature. If spikes occur, the system should be evaluated right once, as drugs can degrade when exposed to excessive temperatures repeatedly.

Automated Dispensing System

Many pharmacies use an automated dispensing technology to increase efficiency and accuracy. These systems typically hold a huge number of individual tablets. The required quantity is determined digitally (or the system might be linked to the pharmacy's internal computer system). The device dispenses the requested quantity into a pill bottle, which is labeled by the technician and verified by the pharmacist. It is critical that the automated system is refilled with the appropriate medication and that the final check is never neglected. If controlled drugs are stored in the automated dispensing system, a second count by a technician or pharmacist is required.

Lot Numbers and Expiration Dates

Every medication and medical supplies at the pharmacy is labeled with a lot number and expiry date. Expiration dates ensure that all pharmaceuticals in the pharmacy are used while they are still useful and can be removed before they expire. The lot number indicates the manufacturer's lot the drug was created in. When a medicine recall occurs, the medications that will be withdrawn are identified by lot number and expiration date. Keeping pharmaceuticals in their original packaging makes it easier to identify which medications to remove from the pharmacy and maintains quality control.

Drug Recalls

Occasionally, errors arise during the manufacturing or development of pharmaceuticals. Contamination with other products, the improper number of materials, or labeling problems are all possible reasons for a recall. In this situation, the FDA or the drug manufacturer will recall the medications if there is a risk linked with their use. When this happens, the pharmacy will get notified. The medication should be removed from the shelves and stored in the pharmacy, clearly labeled as a recalled product. The manufacturer or FDA will provide additional instructions to the pharmacy on medicine return procedures.

Pneumatic Tube System

A pneumatic tube system is a network of tubes and carriers in hospitals and clinics that allows messages and items to be quickly distributed around the facility without the use of human messengers. The object to be delivered is packaged in a padded carrier that snaps shut. The carrier is then placed in its cradle, and a destination is chosen. The carrier moves via the tube system to its destination. Many hospital pharmacies use pneumatic tube systems to carry stat drugs or single dosages to various regions of the hospital. This frees up staff to perform other jobs. Orders can be sent to the pharmacy from the floors using the pneumatic tube system.

The pneumatic tube system should not be used to deliver the following medications:

- Narcotics
- Medications with fragile packaging
- Very expensive medications
- Medications requiring the signature of the recipient
- Chemotherapy

Prescription Not in Stock

Patients occasionally bring prescriptions to the pharmacy that are either not carried by the store or are "temporarily out of stock." Follow your pharmacy's protocol for dealing with such situations, or you can do the following to help the patient:

- If the drug is not an emergency, order it from the distributor and pick it up the next day.
- Check with other branches of your pharmacy to see if you can borrow the medication or if the patient may fill the prescription there.
- Contact competitors to ask if you can borrow the drug or have the patient go there to fill the prescription. The most important thing is to help the patient receive the medication as soon and efficiently as possible.

Stock Rotation

Stock rotation is the practice of using the product with the earliest expiration date first. As fresh inventory arrives, the products on the shelf should be organized so that the product that will expire first is at the front of the shelf, ensuring that it is utilized first. This fulfills two critical functions in pharmacy:

1. It streamlines the process of checking expiry dates. If the product that would expire first is in the front, it is easier to recognize and remove expired product, preventing it from being administered to a patient.
2. Because the product that expires earlier is at the front, it will be used sooner, avoiding it from expiring on the shelf and so lowering waste and total operating costs.

Pharmaceutical Procurement Policies

Pharmaceutical purchase can be a balancing act. Pharmacies must obtain and store a sufficient supply of drugs to treat patients without experiencing shortages. Keeping a surplus of medication may cause it to expire before being utilized, which might cost the pharmacy money to remove. This removal method wastes time and expensive storage space. Procurement policies may differ from pharmacy to pharmacy depending on the needs of the population served and the available storage space. Pharmacy procurement is frequently performed by a professional team comprised of pharmacy, financial, purchasing, and quality control experts.

Par Level and Reorder Level

The terms par level and reorder level refer to stock levels used to determine how much product should be ordered to maintain a service level and when to reorder product. The par level is the amount that should be kept on the shelf at all times. When the product falls below par, it should be reordered. Par levels can vary substantially based on the pharmacy's location and size, population served, and duration between orders. For example, Pharmacy ABC may be a small pharmacy servicing a young clientele; its amlodipine par level could be 300 pills. The par level at Pharmacy XYZ, a larger store in a more retiree-friendly area of town, may be 3000 tablets.

Receiving Inventory

When the order arrives from the shipper, count the boxes to ensure that you received the expected amount. When the boxes are checked in, open each one and match the contents to the packing sheet. This can be done in a variety of ways, depending on the pharmacy's policies. Some pharmacies will ask you to manually check the order. Larger pharmacies that get larger orders may have a scanning system in place that allows you to scan the goods and have the computer compare it to the invoice before adding it to inventory. Some pharmacy orders are processed through a home office, and the inventory is updated after the order is entered into the computer. In this situation, any errors must be manually repaired. Product should be stored promptly to avoid mistakes, storage concerns, and product loss.

Identify Expired or Unsalable Stock

Most pharmacies have a system or process in place to help detect and separate expired or unsalable products. A common technique involves assigning technicians to inspect a certain section of the pharmacy monthly for expired or unsalable drugs. Another system may assign one technician to constantly monitor the pharmacy for expired prescriptions. Every part of the pharmacy must be checked. Even with these protocols in place, it is the responsibility of every staff member to check expiration dates before utilizing any medication to ensure its safety.

Logs

There are numerous logs measuring a wide range of characteristics throughout the pharmacy. Some common ones are:

- Refrigerator and freezer temperatures
- Ambient air temperatures
- Equipment cleaning
- Air cleanliness testing
- Calibration of equipment

These logs are vital and should not be overlooked. Changes in temperature in the pharmacy or refrigerator may jeopardize drug integrity. It is critical to track routine sanitation jobs in order to a) ensure that they are completed by workers and b) demonstrate compliance to certification and inspection agencies. Maintaining accurate and up-to-date records is crucial for providing information during safety audits. They should also be easily available, with every pharmacy employee knowing where to find them.

Pharmacy Billing and Reimbursement

Methods of Payment

A retail pharmacy may accept a variety of payment methods. The pharmacy technician must learn to ring up customers using the cash drawer mechanism specific to their pharmacy. The following payment options are likely to be used:

- Cash
- Personal check
- Third party check (power of attorney)
- Third party payer (usually done via computer)
- Flexible spending accounts
- Credit and debit cards
- Financial assistance cards issued by the state

While some pharmacies utilize pharmacy assistants rather than pharmacy technicians to handle the cash drawers, everyone in the pharmacy should understand how to operate the cash drawer and be able to step up to help if needed.

Third-Party Payer

A third-party payer is an organization that pays for health care services but is not the patient or the medical practitioner. Health insurance, whether private or government-provided, is the most prevalent third-party payer. A patient who pays for their prescriptions through a third party must follow the third party's regulations and procedures, which may include limited access to specific medications and treatments. Most third parties are available through pharmacy computer systems and can provide an approval or denial, as well as the amount covered and the patient's liability at the point of sale. Some providers require patients to pay the retail amount and complete out documents before receiving full reimbursement.

Medicaid and Medicare

Medicaid – Medicaid is a government program that provides health care to persons with low incomes or who fulfill other eligibility requirements. Each state operates its own Medicaid program, with expenditures split between the state and the federal government. Medicaid covers dental treatment as well as a screening program known as Early and Periodic Screening, Diagnostic and Treatment, which aids in the identification and diagnosis of children with medical issues.

Medicare – Medicare is a government program that offers insurance and healthcare to individuals over the age of 65, as well as those with permanent or cognitive disabilities or other qualifying illnesses. Medicare consists of four distinct services. The services offered are:

- Medicare Part A: Hospital Insurance
- Medicare Part B: Medical Insurance
- Medicare Part C: Medicare Advantage Programs
- Medicare Part D: Prescription Drug Program

Denied Medication Claim

Third-party payers may deny medication claims for several reasons. When a claim is dismissed, patients still have options. Some of the possibilities offered include:

- The prescriber can be contacted to prescribe a different drug.
- The patient may opt to pay for the medication out of pocket (though this is not an option if the claim was denied because the refill is too soon).
- The patient may appeal the claim to the insurance company.
- The patient may request a special authorization for the medication.

Third-Party Payer Rejection

A series of minor errors can lead a prescription to be refused by a third-party payer. Many of these errors can be easily detected and remedied by the pharmacy technician. When a prescription is rejected, look for the following potential problems:

- The patient's name doesn't match
- The patient's birthday doesn't match
- The patient's gender doesn't match
- The days' supply is incorrect or unusual for the medication
- The prescription was recently filled at another pharmacy (this could also indicate drug-seeking conduct on the side of the patient).
- The prescription is being refilled too soon
- The number of days' supply exceeds the insurance company's limit.

Some of these errors occur within the insurance business. Errors such as birthdays and genders are common. If this is the case, it may be required to temporarily modify the information in the pharmacy database in order to process the prescription until the insurance company can correct the issue.

Prior Authorization

Before paying for a medicine, certain insurance companies will require prior authorization. This means that the drug is only covered if the patient follows a predetermined set of guidelines. Contact the insurance company and explain why the patient requires the drug and cannot use a formulary replacement. Based on the facts provided, the insurance company will decide whether to cover the drug for the patient. Different insurance companies have different rules, such as who must get authorization and how it should be done.

Formulary

A formulary is an organization's chosen list of pharmaceuticals. An insurance firm, like a hospital, will have a drug formulary. Formularies are typically produced to control expenses and are designed by doctors and pharmacists within the organization. During an inpatient stay, hospitals may convert a patient from a non-formulary drug to an equivalent formulary medication. Insurance companies may request prior authorization or deny coverage for prescriptions that are not on their preferred formulary. Patients who are covered by an insurance company have access to the formulary through the firm's written materials or website. Patients are responsible for understanding the contents of their insurance company's formulary.

Co-Pay

The co-pay is the portion of the payment for which the patient is responsible after the insurance company has made its contribution. Co-pays vary greatly based on the insurance provider, individual prescription plan, and type of medication. Most insurance companies use a tiered approach, with preferred drugs and generics priced lower and non-preferred medications priced higher. In most circumstances, submitting the medication to the insurance company using the online computer system will result in the correct co-pay. Patients are responsible for knowing their insurance company's formulary and tiers.

Register Scanned No Co-Pay Prescription

In some situations, a medication will not require a copay. Most pharmacy systems still require the prescription to be scanned at the register when the patient picks it up. This is done for the following reasons:

- It creates a record in the system of the medication being picked up.
- The prescription must be sold through the system before a patient can sign for it.
- It changes the pharmacy's inventory to reflect the medication being sold.
- Procedures vary from store to store, so follow your pharmacy's policy.

No Co-Pay Prescription

When a patient submits a prescription to their insurance company, it may occasionally result in a $0 co-pay. There are several reasons why a patient may receive a prescription with no co-pay:

- Patients who receive medication assistance from the state frequently have no co- pay.
- Coupon programs provided by the manufacturer will often result in a zero co-pay.
- Some pharmaceutical plans cover certain maintenance drugs completely, resulting in a $0 co-pay.

If the patient expected a zero co-pay, it may be required to contact the insurance company to learn about the firm's policies for particular drug. If you have the time, contacting the insurance company on the patient's behalf is an excellent method to give customer service, but it is ultimately the patient's obligation to understand his or her insurance plan.

Insurance Card

The information offered on insurance company cards varies, but there are a few bits of information that are common to all cards that are required to run the prescription. They are:

- The patient's name
- The member ID (including any additional digits such as -00, -01, etc. These numbers identify the patient's relationship to the subscriber)
- The RXPCN
- The BIN
- The group name or number

The information requested will vary depending on the pharmacy's computer system and the insurance company. Some insurance cards provide information on copays. The reverse of the card normally includes the insurance company's address and phone number, which might be useful if a problem arises.

Insurance Subscriber and Dependents

The insurance subscriber is the individual who holds the insurance policy. If the insurance is provided by an employer, the subscriber is the employee who works for the company. If the insurance was acquired individually, the subscriber is the person who purchased the policy and is responsible for paying the premiums. Dependents are other people who are covered under the policy. Dependents can include:

- Spouse
- Minor children
- Stepchildren
- Children up to age 26 who don't have access to another health insurance plan

Laws vary by state. Check the current coverage laws to see who is eligible as a dependent on health insurance.

Billing Services Procedure

In rare situations, insurance companies will reimburse customers for services rendered. Although patients are generally responsible for this operation, pharmacy technicians can offer assistance and direction.

- Contact the insurance company to learn about their procedure. Some allow reimbursement requests to be submitted online, while others will require paperwork to be completed.
- Confirm that the services are in fact reimbursable.
- Print out receipts or other required proof of services rendered.
- Find the address where the information should be mailed or faxed.

ICD Codes

ICD codes are standardized numerical codes that are used to distinguish between various medical disorders. The acronym ICD stands for International Statistical Classification of Diseases and Related Health Problems. In the pharmacy, ICD codes may be necessary for billing certain prescriptions to insurance companies. Insurance companies may only cover recommended drugs for certain conditions. The ICD code is then sent to the insurance company electronically or as part of a prior authorization request. Doctors may write the ICD code on the prescription, but in most situations, the pharmacist must contact the doctor to obtain the ICD code.

Some samples of ICD codes include:

- 780.30 Seizures NOS

- 733.00 Osteoporosis

- 572.80 Liver disease – hepatic failure

Flexible Spending Account

Many insurance firms provide members with the option of a flexible spending plan or flexible spending account as part of their health insurance package. This option deducts money from the patient's pre-tax income and deposits it into an account that can then be utilized to pay for healthcare-related expenses without incurring taxes. The money must be used within the time frame indicated, or it will disappear. One advantage of a flexible spending account is that it can be used to pay for over-the-counter medications and co-pays. Flexible spending account rules differ, and it is the patient's obligation to understand the restrictions and limitations of his or her flexible spending account.

Products Purchased with a Flexible Spending Account

A flexible spending account can be used to purchase a variety of pharmacy products, but the requirements vary by state and plan. The patient is responsible for understanding which things are covered by his or her plan, while some cards will refuse to pay for unlawful purchases. Some of the products that could be qualified are:

- Over-the-counter drugs used to treat a variety of diseases with a doctor's prescription.

- Diabetes testing supplies, including strips, alcohol wipes, and more

- Syringes for injecting medications

- Bandages and other first-aid necessities

- Other items that would be deductible as medical tax expenses

Pharmacy Information System Usage and Application

Automated Medication-Dispensing Devices

Automated medication dispensing machines are frequently used in hospitals to store pharmaceuticals on the patient care unit, allowing nurses easy access to patients' doses. These technologies also protect patients and medications while preventing drug diversion. These devices keep the medications in a secured cabinet that can only be accessed with a unique identifier and password. More modern devices can employ technology such as fingerprint scanning to authenticate users. The system monitors the doses administered to patients as well as the individuals who access the cabinet. Advanced systems send reports to a central unit, which pharmacy staff can use to verify the state of every unit in the system and decide which ones need to be replenished. Pyxis, Baxter, and McKesson are some of the most common producers of these systems.

FDA Med Watch Program

The FDA MedWatch Program is an online system that allows people to report adverse occurrences related to drugs and other medical items. Both consumers and healthcare providers can submit reports. In addition to major adverse effects, other information needed includes product quality issues, errors in product use, and failures of treatments that are considered therapeutically comparable. Subscribers also receive safety notifications for drugs as they are posted. The goal of this program is to make it easier to report any safety hazards in order to promote consumer safety and swiftly alert the public.

How to Overcome Test Anxiety

Most people become scared just thinking about taking an exam. A test is a significant event that can have long-term consequences for your future, so it's crucial to take it seriously, and it's natural to be concerned about performing well. Anxiety is normal, however it does not necessarily aid with exam taking or should be accepted as a part of life. Anxiety can have a wide range of effects. These effects might be moderate, such as making you feel somewhat uneasy, or severe, such as impairing your ability to focus or recall even minor details.

If you have test anxiety, whether severe or mild, you should know how to overcome it. To learn this, you must first understand what causes exam anxiety.

Causes of Test Anxiety

While we generally think of anxiety as an uncontrollable mental condition, it can be induced by simple, everyday events. One of the most common causes of test anxiety is a lack of proper preparation for the test. This sensation can be caused by a variety of factors, including poor study habits and a lack of organization, but time management is the most typical culprit. Starting to study too late, failing to manage your study time to cover all of the content, or becoming sidetracked while studying will indicate that you are not well prepared for the test. This may lead to cramming the night before, leaving you physically and psychologically weary for the test. Poor time management can lead to tension, despair, and pessimism due to a lack of preparation and uncertainty about how to address it.

Test anxiety is sometimes caused by unresolved fear rather than a lack of preparedness. This could be a previous test failure or low overall test performance. Comparison to others or the pressure to meet expectations can lead to feelings of inadequacy. Anxiety may be caused by concerns about the future—how failing this test may effect your educational and career ambitions. These anxieties are often wholly unjustified, but they can nevertheless have a detrimental impact on your test performance.

Effects of Test Anxiety

Test anxiety is similar to an illness; if not addressed, it will worsen over time. Anxiety causes poor performance, which perpetuates feelings of fear and failure, resulting in poor performance on following examinations. It can progress from slight anxiousness to a debilitating condition. If allowed to grow, test anxiety can have a significant impact on your academic performance and, as a result, your future.

Test anxiety can affect other aspects of your life. Anxiety on tests can develop into anxiety in any stressful setting, and blanking on a test can lead to panic in the workplace.

132

Fortunately, you don't have to let fear dictate your tests and grades. There are several relatively basic actions you can take to overcome your anxiety and operate properly on tests and in everyday life.

Physical Steps for Beating Test Anxiety

While test anxiety is a significant problem, there is good news: it can be overcome. It does not have to limit your ability to think and recall knowledge. While it may take time, you may start taking actions to overcome anxiety today.

The physical symptoms are the first indication that you may be suffering from anxiety, and the first step in treating it is likewise physical. Rest is essential for maintaining a clear and strong mind. If you are fatigued, it is much simpler to succumb to anxiousness. However, if you develop appropriate sleep habits, your body and mind will be prepared to operate optimally, free of the burden of weariness. Furthermore, resting properly improves your ability to remember information, making you more likely to recall the answers when you see the test questions.

Going to bed on time isn't enough to get a decent night's sleep. It's critical to give your brain time to unwind. To avoid overwork, take regular study breaks and avoid studying before bed. Take some time to relax your mind before attempting to relax your body; otherwise, you may have difficulty falling asleep.

Other components of physical health, in addition to sleep, play a vital role in exam preparation. Good diet is essential for proper brain function. Sugary foods and drinks may provide an initial surge of energy, but this is followed by a fall, both physically and emotionally. Instead, nourish your body with protein and vitamin-rich foods.

Additionally, drink plenty of water. Dehydration can cause headaches and weariness, especially if your brain is already stressed by the rigors of the exam. During extensive tests, it's important to stay hydrated. And, if feasible, bring an energy-boosting snack to munch in between parts.

Exercise, like sleep and diet, is a crucial aspect of physical wellness. Maintaining a consistent fitness plan is beneficial, but taking 5-minute study breaks to walk can help get your blood flowing and clear your mind. Exercise also produces endorphins, which contribute to a happy mood and can help with exam anxiety.

When you care for your physical health, you also improve your mental health. If your body is healthy, your mind is much more likely to be so as well. So take some time to rest, replenish your body with nutritious foods and drink, and get as much exercise as possible. Taking these physical steps can strengthen you and make it easier to overcome test anxiety.

Mental Steps for Beating Test Anxiety

Working on the mental part of exam anxiety can be more difficult, but just like the physical side, there are certain actions you can take to overcome it. As previously said, test anxiety frequently arises from a lack of preparation, therefore the apparent remedy is to prepare for the test. While effective studying is crucial for overcoming exam anxiety, it's necessary to also use additional mental strategies.

First, increase your confidence by recalling yourself of earlier successes, such as tests or tasks that you completed well. If you put in as much work as you did for the previous tests, there's no reason you should fail this one. Work hard to prepare, and then trust your preparation.

Second, surround oneself with supportive individuals. It can be beneficial to join a study group, but make sure the folks you're with will promote a positive mindset. Spending time with people that are nervous or cynical can only make you feel more anxious. Look for those who are driven to study hard because they want to succeed, not because they are afraid of failing.

Third, reward yourself. Even without worry, taking a test is physically and psychologically exhausting, so having something to look forward to can be beneficial. Plan an activity for after the test, regardless of the outcome, such as going to the movies or having ice cream.

If you begin to feel apprehensive while taking the test, remind yourself that you know the subject. Visualize passing the test. Then take a few long, soothing breaths before returning to it. Work through the questions carefully yet confidently, knowing that you can succeed.

Developing a healthy mental attitude to test taking will benefit you in other areas of your life. Test anxiety can negatively impact your mental health and possibly lead to despair. It is critical to overcome test anxiety before it manifests itself in other ways.

Study Strategy

Being prepared for the test is essential for overcoming nervousness, but what exactly does it entail? You might study for hours on end and still feel unprepared. You need a test preparation strategy. The following pages detail our recommended measures to help you plan and overcome the obstacle of preparation.

Step 1: Scope Out the Test

Learn everything you can about the structure (multiple choice, essay, etc.) and topics covered on the test. Collect any study materials, course outlines, or sample examinations that are accessible. Knowing what to expect will not only help you prepare, but it will also help you relax during the test.

Step 2: Map Out the Material

Examine the textbook or study guide and take note of how many chapters or parts it has. Then divide these by the amount of time you have. For example, if a book includes 15 chapters and you have five days to study, you should complete three chapters per day. Even better, if you have the time, set aside an extra day at the end for overall review after going over the information thoroughly.

If you have limited time, you may need to prioritize the material. Look over it and make a note of which areas you believe you already understand and which require revisiting.

While studying, go quickly through the known areas and spend more time on the difficult ones. Make a plan to avoid getting lost along the way. Having a detailed strategy also helps you feel more in charge of the study, which reduces anxiety caused by feeling overwhelmed by the quantity to cover.

Step 3: Gather Your Tools

Decide which study approach is best for you. Do you prefer to highlight sections of the text while studying and then go over them again later? Or do you type out vital information? Or is it better to make flashcards that you can carry with you? Assemble your pens, index cards, highlighters, post-it notes, and any other materials you may require so that you are not distracted by getting up to locate something while studying.

Step 4: Create Your Environment

It's critical to avoid distractions while studying. This covers both obvious distractions like visitors and subtle distractions like an uncomfortable chair (or an overly comfy couch that causes you to fall asleep). Create the greatest learning environment possible, including good lighting and a comfortable workspace. If background music helps you focus, turn it on; otherwise, keep the room silent. When taking notes on a computer, avoid distractions such as social media and games. Silence your phone and disable notifications. Keep water handy by to stay hydrated while studying.

Also, consider the optimal time of day to study. Are you at your freshest first thing in the morning? Try to set aside some time to go over the material. Do you have a clearer mind in the afternoon or evening?

Plan your study session then. Another option is to study during the same time of day that you will take the test, so that your brain becomes accustomed to focusing on the information at that time and is ready to focus when the test arrives.

Step 5: Study!

Once you've completed the Diagnostic test at the start of the Exam Prep guide, and completed all of your study preparation, it's time to start studying. Sit down, take a few moments to clear your mind so you can concentrate, and then begin to follow your study plan. Avoid distractions and procrastination. This is your chance to prepare so that you can take the test with confidence. Make the most of your time and maintain focus.

Of course, you do not want to burn out. If you study for too long, you may not recall the material well. Take regular study breaks. For example, taking five minutes out of each hour to walk briskly while breathing deeply and swinging your arms can help keep your mind sharp. When you reach the end of each chapter or section, conduct a quick review. Remind yourself of everything you've learnt and focus on finishing your studies on the last day. Cramming overwhelms your brain with more knowledge than it can process and remember, and when your mind is exhausted from last-minute studying, it may difficult to recall even previously taught information. Furthermore, the urgency of cramming and the strain on your brain lead to anxiousness. You are more likely to arrive at the test feeling unprepared and unable to think clearly.

So don't cram or stay up late the night before the test, even if it's only to go over your notes slowly. Your brain need more rest than it does to review material. In fact, aim to complete your studies by midday or early afternoon the day before the exam. Give your brain the rest of the day to unwind or concentrate on other tasks, and get a decent night's sleep. This will prepare you for the test and improve your remember of previously studied material.

Step 6: Take a practice test

Many courses provide example tests, whether online or in the study materials. This is a great resource for determining whether you have learned the topic as well as preparing for the test format and setting.

Check the test format ahead of time, including the number of questions, type (multiple choice, free answer), and time limit. Then devise a strategy for getting through them. For example, if you have 30 minutes to complete a 60-question examination, your time limit is 30 seconds each question. Spend less time on questions you already know so you can focus more on the difficult ones.

If you have time for multiple practice tests, take the first one open book with no time limit. Work through the questions at your own time and ensure that you completely understand them. Gradually go to taking a test under test conditions: sit at a desk with all study materials stored and set a timer. Pace yourself to ensure that you finish the test with enough time to check your answers.

After each test, double-check your answers. If you missed any questions, make sure you understand why. Did you misread the question (tests often have complex wording)? Have you forgotten the information? Or was it something you hadn't learned? Review any weak points revealed by the practice tests.

Taking these examinations not only improves your grade, but also helps you overcome test anxiety. If you're used to the test settings, you'll be less concerned, and working through tests until you score well will build your confidence. Take the practice tests until you feel comfortable, and then go into the test knowing you're prepared.

Test Tips

On test day, you should be confident since you have prepared thoroughly and are prepared to answer the questions. Aside from preparation, there are various test-taking tactics you can use to improve your results.

First, as previously indicated, get a decent night's sleep the night before the test (or several nights before, if feasible). Instead of studying late at night, go into the test with a fresh, awake mind.

On the day of the test, avoid making too many alterations to your usual routine. A decent breakfast is essential, but if you don't regularly have one, consider a protein bar instead. If you enjoy coffee, feel free to continue drinking it as usual. Just make sure you time it so that the caffeine doesn't run out in the middle of the test. Avoid sugary beverages and drink enough water to stay hydrated without needing to use the restroom 10 minutes into the test. If your test isn't first thing in the morning, try going for a stroll or performing some light exercise to get your blood circulating.

Allow yourself adequate time to prepare, and leave for the test with plenty of time to spare to avoid the stress of rushing to arrive on time. Another reason to arrive early is to get a decent seat. It is beneficial to sit away from doorways and windows, which might be distracting. Find a comfortable seat, gather your supplies, and calm your nerves before the test begins.

When the test begins, look over the instructions attentively, even if you know what to expect. Follow the instructions carefully to prevent making foolish mistakes.

Then start working through the questions, pace yourself as you've practiced. If you're unsure about a response, don't dwell on it and don't allow it undermine your confidence. Either skip it and return later, or eliminate as many incorrect answers as possible and guess from the remaining ones. As you proceed, don't think about these questions; instead, focus on what comes next.

Even if you're confident that the first answer is correct, read all of the options. Keep reading, and you might find a better one. But don't second-guess yourself if you already know the answer. Your gut feeling is typically correct. Don't allow test fear rob you of what you already know.

If you have time at the end of the test (and the structure allows it), go·back and review your answers. Be cautious about making any changes because your first reaction is usually correct, but check to make sure you did not misunderstand any of the questions or accidently mark the wrong response choice. Look over any you missed and make an educated guess.

Finally, exit the test feeling confident. You did your best, so don't waste time thinking about it or wishing you could alter anything. Instead, enjoy your successful completion of this test.

I hope this PTCB exam prep book proves invaluable in your journey towards success.

Thank you for your support and for being part of our community!

All inquiries should be addressed to our email: infoevolitpublishing@gmail.com

Links for your Bonuses

Use the link below to get **5 Practice Tests, 380 Flashcards, a PDF with over 120 pages of Pharmacy Calculations, 790 questions with detailed answers/explanations, and a PDF Manual Review for the PTCB Exam, all totally free.**

Link: *https://payhip.com/b/rQtyR*

QR COODE:

Now for the Best Part!!

You get to help our community by giving this book a review. Many PTCB students, just like you, know how hard it is to find current, concise, and useful information, especially when starting. Not only your review will help them on their journey, but the information you direct them to, might also save their Career!

Do another PTCB student a favor and leave a review talking about the information you found, what you liked about this guide, and how it helped you...even if it's just a sentence or two!

As a token of our appreciation you will also receive a special bonus:

Over 3 hours of PTCB video lessons.

How to leave a review:

Scan the QR Code.

1. Share your thoughts on Amazon.

2. Email a screenshot of **your live** review to **infoevolitpublishing@gmail.com** to claim your **bonus!**

We are deeply appreciative of your review, as it truly makes a difference in our community. Thank you from the bottom of our hearts.

Best of luck on your path to success!

EvoLit Publishing

Made in the USA
Las Vegas, NV
23 October 2024

10413659R00081